LECTURE NC
ANAESTHE

LECTURE NOTES ON
ANAESTHETICS

John N. Lunn
MD, FFARCS
Reader, University of Wales
College of Medicine
Cardiff, Wales

THIRD EDITION

BLACKWELL SCIENTIFIC PUBLICATIONS

OXFORD LONDON EDINBURGH
BOSTON PALO ALTO MELBOURNE

First published 1979
Reprinted 1979
Second edition 1982
Reprinted 1983
Reprinted 1984
German translation 1984
Third edition 1986

Set by Downdell Ltd., Oxford
and printed and bound
in Great Britain by
Billing and Sons Ltd., Worcester

DISTRIBUTORS

USA
  Blackwell Mosby Book Distributors
  11830 Westline Industrial Drive
  St Louis, Missouri 63141

Canada
  The C.V. Mosby Company
  5240 Finch Avenue East,
  Scarborough, Ontario

Australia
  Blackwell Scientific Publications
  (Australia) Pty Ltd
  107 Barry Street
  Carlton, Victoria 3053

British Library
Cataloguing in Publication Data

Lunn, John N.
  Lecture notes on anaesthetics.—
  3rd ed.
  1. Anesthesia
  I. Lunn, John N.
  617´. 96   RD81

  ISBN 0-632-01588-8

Contents

Preface

A lecture to undergraduates is supposed to illuminate a subject from a different point of view although the rudiments of the matter may already be known to the audience. The extent to which these notes do this will be judged by the reader, but that is their aim. In contrast to other texts, this is aimed primarily at the medical student and is designed to inform him about the scientific and clinical background to the modern practice of anaesthesia.

Anaesthesia is a specialty in which many seemingly unconnected items are brought together and that is the reason for the inclusion of the subject in the undergraduate syllabus. The design of a particular syllabus of anaesthetics for undergraduates is often debated by their teachers. This book provides an answer, if not for the teacher, then for the medical student.

The rapid development of the specialty since the 1840s has continued into the 1980s; several drugs have disappeared from use since the last edition was prepared, and a few more have appeared. It is not necessary to refer to drugs which are no longer available for use, but historically important drugs still have a place in Third World countries and are not therefore neglected. Technology has also advanced recently so that improved techniques of monitoring are now almost commonplace, and medical students should be aware of the use of these important devices.

It is a pleasure again to acknowledge current and former students, colleagues, my own teachers for their help and encouragement, and Mrs Margaret Thomas for her secretarial skills.

John Lunn

1. Introduction

This book considers and particularly emphasises those parts of anaesthetics which any doctor may need to know in his professional life. It is not a handbook of practical anaesthesia for the simple anaesthetic. The state of anaesthesia is undeniably complex and a simplified version does not exist. It is therefore not taught. This is not unusual in the undergraduate medical curriculum; for example, there are many simple surgical operations but their performance is not taught by surgeons. The processes which lead to a decision in medicine are more suitable for study than the practical implementation of that decision. It is therefore hoped that the explanations of the many actions of anaesthetics given in this book will help the diligent student.

The study of anaesthesia is a postgraduate one; nevertheless undergraduates need to know something about the subject. Postgraduates spend several months acquiring the rudimentary skills of anaesthesia so it is impossible in the brief period of time available to undergraduates to do more than introduce them to the subject.

Anaesthesia contrasted with other clinical disciplines

Anaesthetics, in common with all other medical practice, is becoming less pragmatic and more scientific. It is rational to make full use of the educational opportunities which this specialty uniquely affords in this particular regard. But the specialty differs from all others to the extent that its practice depends to such a large extent upon team work. It is often stated that surgical operations are best done as a result of cooperation between equal partners and this is undoubtedly true. This is, however, no different from the proper relationship which should exist between laboratory medicine and bedside medicine. Cooperative work between clinicians in the operating room has proved beneficial to patients and, where this exists, everyone benefits.

The practice of anaesthesia involves both diagnosis and therapy but not in the same way as the general practice of medicine. There are fewer diagnoses to be made in anaesthesia than in general medicine but the time available for making the diagnosis is much briefer. Gross haemorrhage is usually apparent to all observers but its rapid treatment can be

1

lifesaving. The effects of undetected air embolus or gross pneumothorax are lethal and their diagnosis must be prompt. There are a number of rarities (for example, malignant hyperpyrexia and the carcinoid syndrome) whose nature and management need to be immediately recalled if the serious complications which may result in a patient's death are to be avoided. Drug interactions and other untoward events have to be recognised promptly for similar reasons. Diagnoses in general medicine or surgery of similar importance are seldom unravelled within a few seconds.

A general anaesthetic is not a therapeutic exercise in the general sense of the term although therapy may be necessary during a surgical operation. No disease is permanently cured by an anaesthetic. Anaesthetists are, however, almost unique in their use of drugs. No other doctor prescribes and regularly *administers* drugs to his patients. It is in this process that one opportunity for an individual demonstration of the scientific method of hypothesis, experiment, observation, and conclusion in medicine can be taken. The evanescent action of some hypnotics, the analgesic action of narcotics, or the reversal of muscle relaxants by an anticholinesterase are three pharmacological examples. The efficacy of fluid, ventilator or oxygen therapy are examples in other fields.

Few other doctors assess, monitor or measure the effect of drug therapy immediately after its administration in quite the same way as does an anaesthetist. The immediacy of his results are before him, and everyone else, to see. It is probable that nearly all patients are pain-free during surgery as a result of the proper administration of drugs and this notable success rate compares very favourably with other drug therapies.

There is another aspect of the work of anaesthetists which is very different from that of other doctors. If a disaster in theatre occurs (fortunately a rare event), an anaesthetist is frequently called upon to explain what has happened immediately both to his surgical colleagues and sometimes to the patient's relatives. This is different from explanations which can be made after a suitable period of reflection and places anaesthetists in a somewhat exposed position. When death occurs in the operating room, or as a direct result of an event there, they cannot hide behind a cloak of 'Well, let's wait and see what this new drug will do'.

The functions of an anaesthetist in hospital have increased greatly in the last twenty years. Involvement in the preoperative and postoperative care of patients led, in addition to their clear expertise in *peroperative* care, to the inevitable extension of the activity of anaesthetists into intensive therapy. The outcome is that there is hardly a clinical department in any hospital today into which an anaesthetist cannot contribute something to the welfare of patients.

Objectives of the undergraduate course in anaesthesia

There are a number of academic objectives in teaching anaesthetics to medical undergraduates which, it is to be hoped, students will achieve during their attachment to anaesthetics. These are that the students should:

> become aware of the role of an anaesthetist and the scope of anaesthesia and intensive care,
>
> understand all aspects of the management of the unconscious patient,
>
> appreciate the implications of intercurrent general medical disease and its therapy in association with surgery and anaesthesia.

A student should also possess some skills at the end of his attachment in anaesthetics and at least be able:

> to maintain the airway of an unconscious patient,
>
> to use appropriate artificial aids to help in the above,
>
> to inflate the lungs of an apnoeic patient with bag and mask,
>
> to assess the general medical condition of a patient prior to anaesthesia; and to suggest relevant management in relation to anaesthesia to improve this where necessary,
>
> to recognise the physical signs of anaesthesia, and to elicit these in a comatose patient,
>
> to perform simple manoeuvres of measurement of pulse, arterial and central venous blood pressure and of artificial ventilation.

2. Preoperative assessment and preparation

Medical assessment prior to general anaesthesia is best performed by an anaesthetist. Other specialists may be able to suggest therapy designed to improve physiological function, but anaesthetists are the appropriate specialists to assess the probable effects of anaesthesia and surgery. Both the patient and the doctors benefit from this.

How does the patient benefit?

A preoperative visit by the patient's anaesthetist is a very important event for that patient. Until this moment any talk with other doctors about an operation has been, to a certain extent, merely hypothetical. When the anaesthetist comes there is usually not much room for further procrastination: the event is imminent. However trivial the surgery may appear to the medical or nursing staff it is not so for the patient. Many events in the latter's life will subsequently be dated by the reference 'that was before (or after) my operation'.

An anaesthetist wants to discover on this visit various medical facts which may or may not influence the conduct of the subsequent operation. The patient in turn needs the opportunity to tell the anaesthetist about his health as a whole. It is unfortunately true that not all surgeons appear to be concerned with anything other than 'their' (surgical) part.

An equally important purpose of the preoperative visit is the establishment of a proper professional relationship between the patient and the anaesthetist. This relationship may form the basis for a contract, which is similar to any other agreement between individuals.

Patients frequently wish to discuss points about their operation with a doctor who is to be closely involved, and welcome the additional chance which the visit offers despite previous explanations by surgical and nursing staff. Confirmation of these may be sought and all groups of staff have to be careful not to contradict one another: it is the author's practice to confine himself solely to those aspects of his own specialty and to refer all surgical matters to others.

A clear but simple description of what will happen whilst the patient is conscious is all that is necessary. Ignorance of the unknown is largely responsible for much natural anxiety and this can be dispelled by knowledge of the proposed procedures. An explanation is welcomed by most patients including children, the latter particularly appreciate a *truthful but simple explanation* of otherwise mysterious events. Of course, the parents should have already attempted this but they seldom have. Furthermore false promises of freedom from pain may need to be counteracted in order that the child is not deceived.

How do the doctors benefit?

Preoperative assessment enables:

> **identification** of those factors which add to the basic risk of anaesthesia and surgery,
>
> **prescription** of therapy to reduce the risk in a particular patient,
>
> **prognosis** about the probable outcome of the operation and the immediate postoperative period to be made on the basis of the history, physical signs, and results of appropriate tests,
>
> **prophylaxis** of postoperative complications to be considered,
>
> **communication** to take place between all members of the operative team.

Details about the proposed operation can be discussed more effectively after the anaesthetist has become acquainted with all aspects associated with the particular patient. Routines may need to be modified or postponement of operation may have to be considered whilst the therapy has time to become effective. All the above functions cannot be fulfilled by conversation between house staff or nurses and anaesthetists over the telephone. Each of these matters will be considered with reference to specific diseases later in this chapter.

The risks of anaesthesia and surgery

Patients do not come into hospital just to have an anaesthetic and the incidence of morbidity and mortality has therefore to be related to surgery. There is very little epidemiological information about the morbidity of anaesthesia and surgery; more is known about mortality.

The commonest cause of death during operation is uncontrollable surgical haemorrhage. Death from anaesthesia is rare. Other causes of death may be accidents, maladroit manipulations, misadventure or negligence. Death may happen after operation as a consequence of one of the above acute events which has been treated successfully in the initial phase but which subsequently results in death. Death may also follow naturally from the illness for which surgery was performed satisfactorily but ineffectually or from some other condition. All deaths under anaesthesia or within 48 hours of surgery are reported to the coroner (Procurator Fiscal in Scotland). This is not for him to apportion blame but so that the public may be reassured that no crime is hidden under the cloak of medicine.

Table 2.1 Comparative figures for two 6-year periods from one town to show decline in hospital mortality rate

	Average annual number of operations	Average annual hospital mortality rate per 1000 operations
1958/1963	9097 (s.e. 276)	27.5 (s.e. 0.9)
1972/1977	17 753 (s.e. 569)	21.5 (s.e. 0.6)

Most statistics about anaesthetic-related mortality refer to deaths in hospital. The figures for one group of hospitals are shown in Table 2.1. The total number of operations performed year by year progressively increased while the figures for hospital *mortality* show a progressive, if slow and somewhat erratic, decline (Fig. 2.1). This decline may of course, be due not merely to improvements in the safety of anaesthesia but to other factors also. There may today be a greater number of relatively trivial operations or procedures for which, in the past, anaesthesia would not have been used, or which were not then fashionable. A significant increase in the amount of surgery undertaken in day-stay patients has occurred: this results in an apparent improvement in hospital mortality figures. It is also possible that surgical patients are less fit than they were and that the effects of advances in anaesthesia are masked when crude mortality statistics are considered.

Fig. 2.2 shows the important effect of the *age* of the patient. It is not surprising that at the extremes of age hospital mortality is increased. Those patients in the lowest age group include those who have surgery for severe congenital abnormalities which are barely compatible with life. At the other extreme, elderly patients with all the physiological effects of ageing may have several intercurrent pathological conditions which combine to increase the risk of anaesthesia.

Fig. 2.2 also shows the *increased mortality rate following emergency* operations compared with that following elective ones. The patients

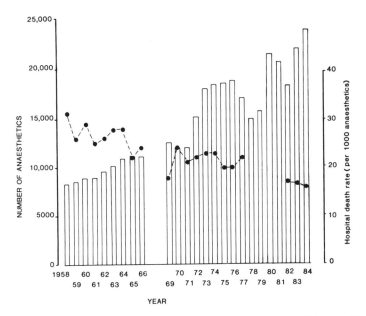

Fig. 2.1. Number of anaesthetics and hospital death rates over 26 years. Vertical columns represent number of anaesthetics; •—•, hospital death rate. (Data from the records system of the Department of Anaesthetics, Cardiff.)

who are untreated for intercurrent medical disease and who require emergency operations are, by definition, less well than those who are prepared for elective procedures. Furthermore, it is probable that more of the surgical procedures themselves are major interventions particularly in old people who, incidentally, should not undergo trivial surgery.

There is also a difference in mortality according to the *gender* of the patient—males have a higher mortality than females; this reflects the known actuarial difference between the sexes and is presumably because fewer minor procedures are performed on men under general anaesthesia.

The *type* of anaesthetic employed tends to reflect the choice of particular agents for poor risk patients, and this so distorts the figures that no conclusion is possible from those that are available.

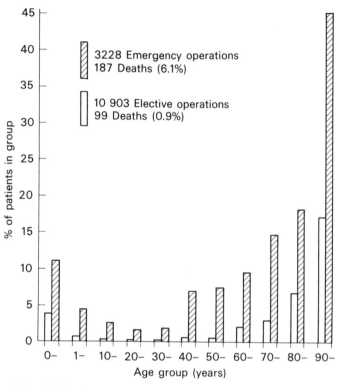

Fig. 2.2.   Relationship between age of patient and hospital mortality. (Data from the records system of the Department of Anaesthetics, Cardiff.)

The overall risk of anaesthesia itself is such that in many situations it is probably one of the safest procedures in medicine. Hazards are still present and it is unwise to imagine that nothing can go wrong nowadays. It can and does. There are many possible dangers: some of these will become apparent later in this book; continuous monitoring of the patient's state is essential (see Chapter 5).

Morbidity after anaesthesia includes many widely diverse symptoms and signs. Nausea, vomiting or retching due to narcotic or anaesthetic drugs is one such, usually evanescent, complication. Bruising of the skin, sore throat, tracheitis, 'hangover', headache and muscle pains (see Chapter 4) are all fairly common, relatively unimportant medically but significant to the patient, and attributable to anaesthesia. The more serious complications of postoperative chest infections, venous thrombosis in the legs or pelvis, or paralytic ileus may be, to some extent at least, affected by the method of anaesthesia. When any complication occurs alone it contributes to morbidity but interactions between several may contribute significantly to mortality.

Elderly patients frequently become disorientated when they are taken away from their familiar surroundings; this disturbance may be exacerbated by anaesthesia and surgery. Powers of mental concentration are commonly reduced for several days in all patients after operation and this is more marked in the elderly. Loss of memory for events within an hour or so of surgery is common.

The preoperative visit

This frequently has to be made in the evening before surgery. It is important that, if there is any doubt about the decision to proceed with surgery, the anaesthetist should be able to see the patient earlier than this; otherwise unnecessary delays and anxiety ensue. When the patient is known to be suffering from serious disease much of the essential information is already available but, because of shortage of time, direct questions, which are normally and properly eschewed in the practice of medicine, are not only allowable but essential. It is to be noted that functional reserve is of greater importance than medical diagnosis. For example the knowledge that a patient is able to walk up stairs without breathlessness is more relevant than the diagnosis of chronic pulmonary fibrosis. The degree of tolerance to exercise indicates the functional reserve. Table 2.2 lists some of these questions. An affirmative answer leads naturally to more specific questions.

Table 2.2   Some of the direct questions which can be used to elicit important information about general health

Have you been in hospital before?
Do you consult your own doctor about any other condition?
Are you allergic to anything?
Are you physically able to do everything you want to?
Have you ever had pain in your chest?
Do you suffer from blackouts or giddiness?
Do you ever become short of breath?
Do you have a cough?
Has anyone in your family ever had trouble with an anaesthetic?

Physical examination usually follows. Particular attention is paid to the state of hydration, the availability of veins, the mobility of the lower jaw and cervical spine, the presence of protuberant, loose, crowned or damaged teeth, all of which are important for technical reasons. The anaesthetist is usually the most senior doctor to examine a surgical patient's chest. It is thus not surprising that unsuspected disease is occasionally revealed.

The place of *screening tests* is slightly controversial. Estimation of haemoglobin, haematocrit, serum electrolytes, blood urea and urine analysis are, in many institutions, regarded as routine. Chest radiography and electrocardiography are discussed later.

Hypoproteinaemia is important since many drugs are bound to proteins and the action of a fixed arbitrary dose may thus be greater in a patient with hypoproteinaemia than in one with normal levels of serum protein. Parenteral nutrition may be indicated to improve the nutritional state of patients who have undergone a period of enforced starvation. Transfusions of albumin have a shortlived effect.

Estimations of plasma cholinesterase (the enzyme responsible for hydrolysis of suxamethonium) or screening for urinary porphyrins, whilst of specific interest to anaesthetists, have not become routine except in a few isolated units. For example, if anaesthesia for electroconvulsive therapy is provided in isolated psychiatric hospitals it is useful to know in advance that the patient is able to hydrolyse suxamethonium normally. Patients with acute intermittent porphyria occasionally present with psychiatric symptoms, and again, rather than precipitate a demyelination crisis with tragic effects, a simple laboratory test can be used to screen for this condition.

Intercurrent medical disease and anaesthesia

The account which follows is not intended to be comprehensive. A few diseases which present as common problems are discussed. The few rarities are mentioned merely to illustrate the importance of proper communication between specialists. The role of a specialist physician called in consultation is not to offer prognostic opinions about anaesthesia but to help ensure that patients are in the best possible state to withstand the effects of anaesthesia and surgery and that no other therapy is indicated.

Cardiovascular disease

Ischaemic heart disease

Patients with ischaemic heart disease present serious risks for anaesthesia and surgery. The functional cardiac reserve is reduced to below that regarded as normal for the patient's age. If symptoms of heart disease exist an electrocardiograph should be performed and a chest radiograph obtained. This should be routine for all patients over 40 years, even in the absence of symptoms.

The symptom of *angina pectoris* and, in particular, the stimulus which provokes it, is a very important qualitative guide. Angina at rest provoked by mental stress is more serious than angina which is provoked by exertion in cold weather. The symptom indicates inadequate myocardial blood flow in response to increased requirements.

A history of *myocardial infarction* is also relatively serious. If the patient has a normal exercise tolerance without breathlessness or angina, and is free from complications of myocardial infarction, the risk is less than if these symptoms and signs are present. When the interval between the infarction and the operation is less than three months, the reinfarction rate becomes about 40%. This postoperative infarction, like any other repeat infarction, is more likely to be fatal. The incidence of further infarction postoperatively declines as the interval between the first infarct and the operation lengthens until, at about two to three years, the incidence becomes the same as that for the general population. Therefore, if recent infarction has occurred, it is clearly beneficial to delay the operation if possible, and it is not in the patient's interest for cosmetic or elective procedures to be performed shortly after coronary occlusion.

There is not much knowledge about prophylaxis against postoperative infarction, but adequate analgesia with consequent freedom from stress would seem to be an important matter.

Oxygen therapy and electrocardiographic monitoring should be continued in high-risk patients until the third or fourth day, since this is the commonest period during which postoperative infarction occurs.

Dysrhythmias, atrial fibrillation, partial or complete heart block, left bundle branch block, or ventricular ectopics may indicate ischaemic heart disease. Pre-existing dysrhythmias may be aggravated by (inadvertent) hypoxia, hypercapnia, changes of hydrogen ion activity, or electrolyte disturbances. Anaesthetic agents sensitize the heart to the action of catecholamines which are released in these circumstances; haemodynamic deterioration may then develop and the dysrhythmia change from a relatively benign one into ventricular tachycardia or fibrillation. Antidysrhythmic therapy or temporary artificial pacing may be required preoperatively if surgery is essential: guidance may need to be sought from a cardiac physician.

Cardiac failure

Patients in cardiac failure cannot increase their cardiac output in response to metabolic requirements, organ perfusion is poor (including that of the myocardium) and they are more prone to postoperative venous thrombosis and chest infection. Uptake of inhaled gases and vapours is impaired. Surgery, other than that necessary to save life, should not be performed on patients with untreated cardiac failure. The briefest delay allows emergency therapy to be commenced and even a few hours spent preoperatively improves the otherwise slender chance of patient survival.

When a patient is suffering from chronic heart failure and has been treated, it is important to be sure that improvement in cardiac function cannot be achieved by more bed rest, and/or a change of diuretics or antidysrhythmic therapy: an expert opinion about this matter should be sought.

There are occasions, for example before thoracotomy in the elderly, where prophylactic digitalis may be recommended in order to improve cardiac function in patients who, though not decompensated, are at real risk from becoming so as a result of fluid loss and replacement or electrolyte changes in association with surgery or the onset of atrial fibrillation.

Hypertension

Antihypertensive therapy should be continued throughout the operative period. The dangers of rebound hypertension, with the consequent risk of a cerebrovascular catastrophe following withdrawal, far outweigh any disadvantages of continuing therapy. For example, the incidence of dysrhythmias and myocardial hypoxia during laryngoscopy and intubation is substantially lower in those patients who are maintained on their therapy with beta adrenergic blocking agents than in those who are not. The hypoxic damage to the myocardium is permanent although the ECG tracing returns to normal. Hypertension, although transient, may result in permanent cerebral damage from cerebral haemorrhage. Furthermore, the cardiovascular system is more stable throughout anaesthesia and surgery in treated than untreated hypertensive patients.

Congenital heart disease

Asymptomatic patients are at no great risk from the anaesthetic (in the absence of shunt reversal following systemic hypotension or misapplied intermittent positive pressure ventilation) but prophylaxis against bacterial endocarditis must always be considered. Appropriate antibiotic therapy is essential in dental, colonic, rectal or gynaecological surgery. Anticoagulation in patients with prosthetic valves must be continued until just before surgery, and is more conveniently provided by heparin than by other anticoagulants, since this can be reversed readily with protamine sulphate.

Respiratory disease

Disease of the airways and the lungs may affect oxygenation, carbon dioxide elimination, uptake of inhaled gases and cause an increase in the incidence of postoperative chest infections. Severe life-threatening bronchospasm may occasionally be precipitated in asthmatics or in nicotine addicts, but in general it is remarkable how rarely respiratory disability seriously interferes with the conduct of anaesthesia itself. This is plainly the result of the growth of proper preoperative screening, postponement and prophylaxis, combined with care in the choice of method of anaesthesia. Effective antibiotics, analgesia and physiotherapy in the postoperative period are essential in the prevention and treatment of postoperative pneumonia.

Coryza

It is usual to postpone elective surgery for any patient with an upper respiratory tract infection since it is reasoned that the effect of sedative drugs and atropine, and the reduction in immunological responses associated with general anaesthesia, must increase the risk of postoperative chest infections. Some patients reveal that an upper respiratory tract infection is always followed by bronchitis in their particular experience. It is foolhardy to continue with anything but life-saving surgery in such patients: each attack of bronchitis leaves additional permanent scars which cause further functional respiratory impairment. Postoperative pain inhibits coughing, so that clearance of secretions may be ineffective. This scheme of management of upper respiratory tract infections is based on somewhat slender evidence but the dilemma will not be easily resolved except by a proper randomized clinical trial. The group of patients, children, in whom coryza is so common and where the postponement of surgery is frequent, is just that group in which study is ethically extremely difficult. It is, however, rational to postpone operation because concomitant swelling of mucous membranes, adenoidal and tonsillar tissue, together with the increased volume of secretions are such that the patency of the airway is easily jeopardized when the child is unconscious. Airway reflexes are much more brisk, and coughing and laryngospasm are common during general anaesthesia in small children with colds.

Chronic respiratory disease

This term includes a number of specific disease processes which have common functional effects. Patients with chronic bronchitis, emphysema, pneumoconiosis or asthma are frequently found in surgical wards. There are two questions posed by the problems which these patients present. Firstly, can the patient be anaesthetized safely? The commonest answer to this is 'Yes' because most anaesthetists know from their experience that this is so. Secondly, and much more importantly, will either the anaesthetic or the proposed surgical procedures seriously and permanently impair respiratory function postoperatively? Temporary impairment as a result of pain can be lessened either by regional analgesic techniques (see Chapter 4) and physiotherapy, or by automatic ventilation (see Chapter 7). Permanent impairment may follow the removal of part of a lung and the benefits of such surgery must be weighed against the disadvantages of reduced respiratory function.

A clinical history and physical examination reveals the type of respiratory impairment but tests of lung function are required to quantitate this.

Chest X-rays should be taken to establish a baseline in any patient with respiratory symptoms and signs and probably in all other patients over the age of forty years to exclude the presence of lung disease. On other occasions routine chest radiography in fit patients as part of a screening process is almost certainly a waste of resources. *Sputum* should be cultured and the sensitivity to antibiotics of any growth tested.

Vital capacity and the *timed force expiratory volume* (FEV) should be related to reference values for patients of the same gender and height. *Peak flow rate* measurement is commonly employed for, and by, asthmatics to help in the management of bronchodilator therapy but random measurements are not so informative as are those of vital capacity and forced expiratory volume. Reduction of both these values is commonly found although each test can be used separately to identify elements of obstructive or restrictive lung disease. The response to bronchodilators can be assessed by improvements in the FEV, and this is a useful guide to treatment if an asthmatic element in the airways obstruction is suspected.

These tests demonstrate the extent of the *ventilatory reserve*. The prediction of the need for postoperative automatic ventilation can rationally be based on the results of these tests. Less severe respiratory impairment revealed by the tests preoperatively indicates that postoperatively the patient's cough may be ineffective. It is necessary to be able to take a deep breath (vital capacity) in order to exhale rapidly enough (forced expiratory time) to cause mucus to be dislodged and expelled from the respiratory tract.

Complex tests of respiratory function are seldom required as part of preoperative screening though they may be very useful in the differentiation of the causes of dyspnoea.

Arterial blood gas analysis should be performed on patients whose vital capacity is less than 60% of the reference value, or whose one-second forced expiratory volume ($FEV_{1.0}$) is less than 60% of the measured vital capacity. The ventilatory reserve in these patients is close to a critical level and the additional information may be of prognostic or postoperative importance.

Preoperative management: patients with a productive cough are probably helped by *physiotherapy*. This is particularly so in those rare patients with bronchiectasis in whom supervised postural drainage is of obvious benefit. *Prophylactic antibiotics* are not indicated except in prosthetic surgery. If there is a seasonal, allergic element in the aetiology of the bronchospasm it is sensible to delay non-urgent surgery until that season has passed; otherwise the effective antihistamine or bronchodilator should be prescribed.

Smoking must be stopped, if possible for several days. The benefit of an improved airways resistance and surfactant turnover rate is achieved over this period. A briefer period of abstinence than this may be less beneficial both psychologically and physically. Nevertheless a few patients may be able to break their addiction subsequently.

Chronic sinusitis should be treated before elective major thoracic or abdominal surgery. It is a common cause of postoperative respiratory complications. Acute bronchitis should be treated before surgery.

It is extremely rare for patients in *respiratory failure* to require elective surgery. Patients who are receiving automatic ventilation for intercurrent respiratory failure present no particular problem for anaesthesia when, for example, tracheostomy is required.

Many patients with serious *respiratory impairment* require anaesthesia for surgery. Ideally, this surgery should be undertaken in institutions where there are proper facilities for thorough assessment preoperatively and for intensive therapy postoperatively. (The question of the choice of an appropriate anaesthetic technique is considered in Chapter 6.)

Most patients with *minor impairment* of respiratory function are managed in a manner no different from a normal patient. Increased reactivity of the bronchial musculature is a relative contraindication to tracheal intubation.

Diabetes mellitus

This condition is properly managed by a team which includes a physician interested in the management of diabetic patients. Operations upon diabetics can be safely conducted provided that a few simple arrangements are agreed.

Anaesthesia in normal subjects is associated with a modest rise in blood sugar (less than 5 mmol/litre) which is due to a reduction in the circulating level of insulin and an increase in circulating catecholamines. Two anaesthetic agents of almost historical interest only, ether and cyclopropane, specifically increase the blood sugar but halothane, or narcotic supplemented nitrous oxide anaesthesia with muscle paralysis and controlled ventilation of the lungs, have no significant effects.

Unstable diabetics should not be anaesthetized for elective surgery unless the surgical condition (e.g. infection in a diabetic's foot) is the cause of the instability. Ketoacidosis must be treated urgently before anaesthesia, since metabolic acidosis has serious effects upon cardiac function and upon the action of drugs. The customary metabolic derangements of anaesthesia and surgery are additive.

Hyperglycaemia in *mature-onset* diabetes may be controlled by oral antidiabetic tablets and diet alone. Oral hypoglycaemic tablets are withheld on the day of operation and a blood sugar estimation obtained preoperatively. Glucose is given intravenously if required. The long half-life of chlorpropamide and glibenclamide should be noted, because hypoglycaemia can occur later if glucose is not administered. Postoperatively, the blood sugar estimation must be repeated in order to determine the need for further intravenous glucose. If prolonged ileus is anticipated it may be necessary to start temporary management with soluble insulin.

Insulin-dependent diabetics require both insulin and glucose during anaesthesia and surgery. If possible, operations should be performed in the morning, and soluble insulin is often substituted for the long-acting drugs to facilitate management. A 5% dextrose infusion is started in the morning and half the patient's usual insulin requirement is given; a blood sugar estimation is performed immediately before surgery as a check.

Additional glucose or insulin may be required during surgery and this is indicated by the results of repeat estimations of blood sugar or by means of Dextrostix papers. Postoperatively an appropriate sliding scale of insulin dosage against urinary glucose levels, combined with occasional blood sugar estimations, is used to guide therapy. This scale is determined for the individual patient.

Obesity

Simple obesity exists when more than 25% of body weight in males (30% in females) is fat. Obesity is one cause of restrictive lung disease, and is associated with diabetes mellitus and hypertension.

Gross simple obesity should not be confused with cardiorespiratory failure of obesity, which occurs in less than 10% of obese people. This occurrence is marked by alveolar hypoventilation from which stem the other indicators of the syndrome: florid or cyanotic facies, systemic and pulmonary hypertension and hypertensive heart disease.

Most surgeons, not to say anaesthetists, would prefer to delay operation in obese subjects wherever possible until sufficient weight has been lost. It should be understood that a serious risk of death exists whenever a grossly obese patient is anaesthetized. This risk arises because of difficulty with the airway, inaccessible veins, poor ventilatory effort, difficult and prolonged surgery, increased risk of wound infection, venous thrombosis and pulmonary embolism. It is worth noting that not only is the volume of gastric contents in starving obese patients increased but also that these contents are more acid. Regurgitation of stomach contents can happen readily owing to the higher incidence of hiatus hernia in obese patients and therefore prophylaxis, for example with an alkali, is desirable.

Skeletal disease

Difficulty may be experienced in the maintenance of the airway or during intubation because of deformity or reduced mobility of the cervical spine, or the involvement of the temporomandibular joints. The patient may complain of hoarseness or progressive weakness of voice when the cricoarytenoid joints are involved. Coughing may thus be impaired.

Arthritic changes in the elbow or wrist joints may interfere with access for venepuncture, and the skin of patients with rheumatoid arthritis is frequently thin.

Anaemia is a common feature in rhematoid arthritis; it may be aggravated by gastrointestinal blood loss following the use of some analgesic drugs or by bleeding caused by drug-induced thrombocytopenia. This anaemia may require treatment prior to surgery and, since it is refractory to any other therapy, blood transfusion is used.

Particular care is necessary with these patients because some joints are less well protected from extreme movements as a result of the reduction in muscle tone due to anaesthesia. Cervical subluxation is a potential result of manipulation of the neck prior to tracheal intubation in patients with rheumatoid arthritis. Adequate soft support needs to be provided by pillows, and care must be taken to avoid positions which were. impossible for the patient to achieve spontaneously. Excessive strain upon ligamentous supports may result in painful joints after the operation. The patient must be encouraged to resume the fullest possible activity as soon as possible after operation so that previously mobile joints do not become immobile. A few operations require unnatural postures to be adopted (lithotomy, prone or Mohammedan praying position) and particular care should be taken in these circumstances.

The possibility of steroid suppression of the adrenals must be considered if these drugs have been used recently (see page 21).

Liver disease

Severe liver failure must be present before the metabolism of drugs is affected to a notable extent; the number of enzymes present in the reduced mass of liver cells is increased and therefore metabolism is not affected at first. Analgesic and sedative drugs may have a prolonged action because brain metabolism is also altered in liver disease.

Anaesthesia in patients with jaundice carries two significant risks. Haemorrhage from prothrombin deficiency is one: vitamin K is given prophylactically. The second risk is renal failure; bilirubin accumulates in the renal tubules and, unless a diuresis is maintained, can cause renal failure. Mannitol is commonly given throughout the operative period to encourage urine flow.

Anaemia

The mechanisms which compensate for the effects of chronic anaemia may be upset by anaesthesia and surgery, particularly if haemorrhage occurs. Increased ventilation and increased cardiac output may both be abolished by anaesthesia, but neither the reduced viscosity of blood nor the increased delivery of oxygen at the tissues, (caused by the increased amounts of 2-3 diphosphoglycerate in anaemia) are affected. Clearly haemorrhage may reduce the amount of circulating haemoglobin to a critical level. Theoretically the amount of oxygen available is reduced if acute changes in cardiac output or oxygen saturation occur, and Table 2.3 shows some worked examples of the equation of oxygen availability. The basal level of oxygen uptake in a conscious subject is about 250 ml per minute. It is presumed that available oxygen should not be permitted to fall below this figure.

There is no evidence that anaemia *per se* affects the outcome of surgery in terms of mortality, complications or hospital stay, but it is impossible to guarantee freedom from accidents, including reduced cardiac output and hypoxaemia, and therefore it is usually suggested that elective surgical patients should have a preoperative haemoglobin level of about 10 g/100 ml.

The management of any anaemic patient prior to surgery includes the diagnosis of the cause of the anaemia and particularly, does *not* include blood transfusions merely in order to satisfy arbitrary criteria of acceptability for anaesthesia. Blood transfusion is, however, sometimes indicated and this is best administered at least 48 hours prior to surgery so

Table 2.3 The theoretical equation of oxygen availability

Available oxygen or oxygen flux (Av.O$_2$)

$$= \frac{\text{Cardiac}}{\text{output}} \times \frac{\text{Haemoglobin}}{\text{concentration}} \times \frac{\text{Oxyhaemoglobin}}{\text{saturation}} \times \frac{\text{Haemoglobin}}{\text{carrying capacity}}$$

For a (theoretically normal) subject

$$= 5000 \times \frac{15}{100} \times \frac{100}{100} \times 1.34 \quad \left(\frac{\text{ml}}{\text{min}} \times \frac{\text{g}}{\text{ml}} \times \frac{100}{100} \times \frac{\text{ml}}{\text{g}} \right)$$

$$\text{(i.e. ml/min)}$$

Av.O$_2 \simeq 1000$ ml O$_2$/min.
For a moderately anaemic but otherwise normal subject,
Av.O$_2 \simeq 770$ ml O$_2$/min

If cardiac output were then to be halved (haemorrhage, overdose of anaesthetic
etc.)
Av.O$_2 \simeq 380$ ml O$_2$/min

If oxygen haemoglobin saturation were then also to be reduced to 75%
Av.O$_2 \simeq 285$ ml O$_2$/min.

---

that the fluid and electrolyte load can be redistributed and excreted. The practice of transfusion during the night before surgery is not only inhumane but also bad applied physiology. It is doubtful whether oxygen carriage is immediately improved, since the transfused blood contains less 2–3 diphosphoglycerate than normal; the increased blood volume and electrolyte load may do more harm than the red cells do good.

Sickle cell disease should be suspected in every patient of Negro origin, or from the Middle East or the Mediterranean. Enquiry should be made about the symptoms of unexplained recurrent abdominal or joint pains. Screening for sickle cell trait is now simplified by use of the Sickledex test. If a patient is positive to this test and is anaemic a full haematological assessment is required, and the risk of anaesthesia and surgery should be carefully considered. Acidosis, dehydration and hypoxia cause sickling; these cannot with absolute certainty always be prevented and general anaesthesia is therefore avoided wherever possible. Local anaesthesia is not without risk either. Sickle cell trait itself does not present any additional risk.

Current drug intake

It is not uncommon for questions about drug intake to reveal unsuspected and important medication. The list of theoretical interactions between anaesthetic drugs and others is quite long but, it must be admitted, only a few commonly cause problems.

Steroid therapy is prescribed for a large number of conditions. The recipients are at risk from acute cardiovascular collapse which occurs during surgery. The precise cause is neither known nor is it possible to relate plasma cortisol levels to the incidence of hypotension. If treatment is, or has been, in progress for two weeks or more at the time of operation, supplementary cover for the immediate period must be provided. Intramuscular and intravenous hydrocortisone should be used one day before and on the day of operation. This dose is then gradually reduced over the next two to three days to the maintenance regimen. If otherwise unexplained hypotension occurs during or after the procedure larger doses of hydrocortisone are given intravenously.

The use of oestrogen containing *contraceptive pills* should be stopped one month before major elective surgery, since the relative risk of deep vein thrombosis is approximately twice that of non users. If this is not possible, active prophylaxis with low dose subcutaneous heparin and/or dextran infusions should be provided.

Monoamine oxidase inhibitors are less commonly used than formerly for the treatment of endogenous depression. There are two dangerous interactions between these agents and drugs which are used in association with surgery. Firstly, an excessive response to exogenous catecholamines may occur, for example following the administration of indirectly acting vasoconstrictors, because excessive amounts of noradrenaline may accumulate. This does not occur when adrenaline is added as a vasoconstrictor to local analgesic drugs. Secondly, the metabolism of pethidine by microsomal enzymes of the liver is inhibited by these drugs, and profound respiratory depression with either hypertension or hypotension may occur. A similar reaction may follow the use of morphine. These interactions may arise up to 14 days after the withdrawal of the monoamine oxidase inhibitors.

An allergic response to drugs or food should be carefully noted, since serious allergic phenomena in response to anaesthetic drugs tend to be noticed in patients who are allergic to other substances. Similar attention should be paid to the report of 'sensitivity' to particular drugs. These responses are not always serious and may be limited merely to an urticarial rash. However, occasionally, a fully anaphylactic response (severe bronchospasm, widespread oedema and hypotension) occurs under anaesthesia. Prompt treatment is necessary with intravenous hydrocortisone and intravenous fluids.

The effect of the social use of *alcohol* is a useful comparator in the description of some drug effects. If intake is considerable and habitual, weight-related doses of central depressant drugs may be less effective than normal. Excessive intake of alcohol may affect hepatic destruction of drugs: all sedative and narcotic drugs are contraindicated in severe liver failure.

Previous anaesthetic history

Many patients have had previous surgery and their memories of any unpleasant effects are remarkably good. Postoperative *nausea* and *vomiting* is commonly not due to anaesthetic drugs but to concurrently administered narcotic analgesics. Both symptoms are also stated to be more common following certain operations, such as dilatation and curettage. Antiemetics (cyclizine, droperidol, metoclopramide or perphenazine) should be prescribed in the attempt to prevent this distressing complaint, but these drugs are not always effective in the patient whose vomiting is habitual after anaesthesia. *Headache* is also a common after-effect which should be treated with mild analgesics: it is particularly common after halothane anaesthesia and may be related to the increased cerebral blood flow which is an effect of this drug.

Patients are occasionally told that they were '*sensitive* to the anaesthetic'. It is impossible to know in the absence of a written record what this may have meant, but it is foolhardy to ignore the information. An effort should be made to discover the reason for this warning. A particular form of this report is the statement that a close blood relative died under anaesthesia. This is clearly a source of considerable anxiety and again, some effort should be made to find out the causes of the disaster without alarm to the patient. There are a few hereditary or familial conditions which have serious anaesthetic implications (malignant hyperpyrexia, dystrophia myotonica, porphyria, variations in plasma cholinesterase).

A history of *awareness* during a previous procedure is another rare event but it must be taken seriously. A particular effort to minimize the anxiety which this would cause is essential.

If anaesthesia needs to be *repeated* at brief intervals it is probably best to use different agents on each occasion. It is certainly true that there is an association between the occurrence of jaundice postoperatively and repeated anaesthesia (within four weeks) with halothane. The cause of the affliction is unknown but if severe liver failure develops it is often fatal.

Preoperative preparation for elective surgery

Patients whose operations are to be performed in the morning are starved of food and fluid from the previous evening. If the operation is to be in the afternoon they are often allowed a 'light' breakfast. Intercurrent drug therapy is administered parenterally although if tablets can be swallowed with the aid of a few millilitres of water this is usually acceptable.

The patient is labelled with name, address and hospital number so that, particularly in a large operating suite, confusion about the identity of a patient can be avoided. Nurses encourage patients to take the last opportunity of a bath before operation because this may be impossible for a few days afterwards. Standard hospital operating gowns are worn by all patients. Dentures, jewellery and make-up are usually removed: the former for safe storage and the latter to enable natural colours to be seen readily by observers. Small dental plates are particularly liable to cause airway obstruction if they become dislodged. Metallic jewellery may come into contact with metal parts of the operating table; in the event of faulty earthing, of diathermy machines for example, these contacts may be the site of small burns.

3. Principles of anaesthetic apparatus

Anaesthetic drugs are either inhaled or administered by injection. Preparation and accurate administration of inhaled drugs are just as important as for injected ones. *Study of the principles of the apparatus* for the former *is worthwhile because the lessons can be applied in other fields* but detailed knowledge is not necessary for medical students.

The anaesthetic machine

There are several different designs of machine in use but the general appearance is similar to that in Fig. 3.1.

Gases are metered through flowmeters, via vaporizers for volatile agents, to breathing systems for attachment to the patient.

Gases

Gases are stored under pressure in cylinders: these may be located peripherally at the site of use or kept centrally in a bank of large cylinders which supplies a pipeline for distribution of gas throughout the hospital. A liquid oxygen supply is used in large installations because this is more economical than large banks of cylinders.

Non-interchangeable connections for special gases are used between pipeline outlets and anaesthetic machines or wall-mounted flow meters. Connections between cylinders and anaesthetic machines are similarly protected from cross-connection by the pin-index system which prevents the accidental attachment of an inappropriate cylinder.

The contents gauge of an oxygen cylinder indicates the pressure within, and this is directly proportional to the volume of gas which remains in the cylinder in accord with Boyle's law (see Appendix). Nitrous oxide exists as a liquid when it is stored at increased pressure in cylinders: about three-quarters of a full cylinder is liquid. The pressure gauge does not therefore reflect the volume which remains in the cylinder until all the liquid nitrous oxide is exhausted.

Gas flows as a result of a pressure gradient between two points. The very high pressure within a gas cylinder (nitrous oxide: 51 atmospheres (*ca* 5100 kPa); oxygen: 120 atmospheres (*ca* 12 000 kPa)) must be

24

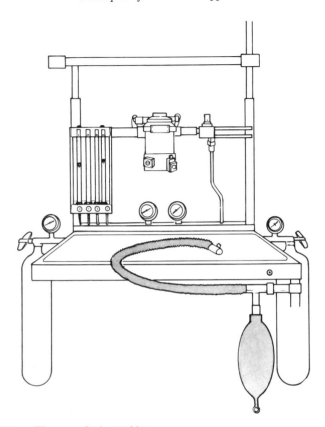

Fig. 3.1. The anaesthetic machine.

reduced. This high pressure would not only be dangerous but also it would be necessary continually to adjust a high resistance in the outflow of the gas to ensure constant flow.

Pressure reduction at the first stage is achieved by means of reducing valves; in principle these function by the conversion of the high pressure, which acts over a small cross-sectional area, to a low pressure which acts over a large area. In the absence of downstream resistance to flow, reduction from 4 atmospheres (*ca* 400 kPa) to just above atmospheric pressure (*ca* 100 kPa) occurs at the needle valve which controls the gas flow through the flow meter.

Flow meters (Fig. 3.2) are the means whereby correct concentrations of gases are prepared for administration to patients. There are several

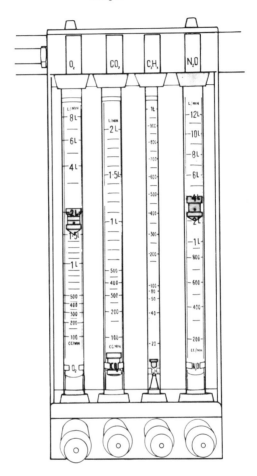

Fig. 3.2.   A bank of four flow meters. Note that the reading is made at the top of the bobbin which is freely rotating, and that the scales of flow meters for different gases are themselves different.

types which indicate volume flow rate of continuously flowing gas. The tubes have an internal diameter which is wider at the top of the tube than at the bottom. In the commonest type of flow meter, the Rotameter, a light alloy bobbin floats in the stream of gas. Its top margin is aligned, without parallax, with the scale on the side of the tube in order to make a reading. The bobbin must be seen to rotate freely.

Flow meters on anaesthetic machines have an overall accuracy of ± 5% provided that they are used properly. They must be:
    used for the specific gas for which they were calibrated,
    clean,
    mounted vertically,
    dry,
    free from static electrical charges,
    free from back pressure.

If these precautions are observed flow meters give accurate readings; if they are not, very serious errors are possible and dangerously hypoxic mixtures can be delivered. The same is true of the use of wall-mounted flow meters in wards. The design of the latter is similar to that of those used on anaesthetic machines, except that the bobbins are round and plastic. The maximum output of these flow meters is about 15 litres/min, although the scale usually extends only to 10 litres/min.

Anaesthetic machines have a bypass for oxygen so that 100% O_2 may be delivered directly, at a high flow rate, at a point in the breathing system beyond the flow meters and vaporizers. Some machines are also equipped with safety blow-off valves (set at 5 lb/in^2 *ca* 35 kPa) to protect the flow meters and other apparatus which may be attached. There are also devices to indicate when a cylinder is empty or that the pipeline supply has failed. These may simultaneously dump nitrous oxide to the atmosphere and enable the patient to breathe air.

Vapours

The devices in which vaporization of liquid anaesthetics takes place are called vaporizers. They are designed to deliver known concentrations of anaesthetic vapours.

History

In the earliest days of anaesthesia the importance and convenience of vaporizers for use during anaesthesia were appreciated. The ideas which inventors incorporated into their design have not altered today, although there are some additional features in modern vaporizers. Diethyl ether, the agent in use at the time, in common with other liquids cools when it is vaporized. The consumption of the heat of vaporization in turn reduces vaporization because the saturated vapour pressure is temperature dependent. Thus the concentration which issues from a simple vaporizer also progressively declines. If heat is supplied continually to the vaporizing chamber cooling is prevented and a more nearly constant concentration is emitted. John Snow's (1812-1858) version was therefore made of copper and the ether container was itself immersed in hot water. The effective surface area of the vaporizer exposed to the heat was increased by the spiral design of the container for the ether. Joseph Clover (1825-1882) later added a system in his design whereby the concentration of ether could be varied.

The concentration of ether which these vaporizers delivered was dependent upon the ventilation of the patient. Hyperventilation led to increased vaporization and vice versa. Such compensation for changes in flow rate of air across the ether was also required, but was not achieved until later.

Modern vaporizers

Vaporizers are usually mounted close to flow meters on anaesthetic machines; constant flows of anaesthetic gas pass through them. Draw-over vaporizers (in which gas is drawn over the liquid by the patient's efforts) are less commonly used in hospital for general anaesthesia, but they are used in field conditions and in obstetric units for self-administered analgesia. Performance specifications state the limits of ventilation between which repeatable concentrations are provided by the apparatus.

The effects of changes in ambient temperature or of the temperature of the liquid anaesthetic are prevented by thermocompensatory devices. One design of these is a bimetallic strip. The two metals of the strip expand differently in response to an increase in temperature, and therefore the strip bends. This either varies the proportion of fresh gas which comes into contact with the liquid anaesthetic, or varies the dilution of saturated vapour with gas that has bypassed the vaporizing chamber. Many vaporizers are made of metal which acts as a reservoir of heat, and this helps to maintain the liquid anaesthetic at room temperature. The process of vaporization is encouraged by causing the liquid to be spread over a large surface area by capillary attraction of the liquid over cloth, canvas or metal wicks. Resistance downstream from a vaporizer can, particularly if intermittent, allow gas to be exposed twice to the liquid anaesthetic. This causes a high concentration of anaesthetic to be delivered to the patient. One-way valves and a resistance are often incorporated within a vaporizer to minimize this effect. Concentrations of vapour are thus accurately prepared and are repeatable over a wide range of fresh gas flow and ambient temperatures. Very high or very low barometric pressures (hyperbaric chambers or high altitude) alter the performance. There is a noninterchangeable filling system for one series of commercial vaporizers to prevent the accidental introduction of the incorrect agent.

The above examples of some features of modern vaporizers are sufficient to show that even today their design depends on the early principles worked out by the pioneers of anaesthesia in the United Kingdom.

Breathing systems

There are several, superficially very different, breathing systems used in anaesthetic practice. The detailed variations in design and performance are important to anaesthetists because they have practical consequences, but only the principles are important to undergraduates. One of the commoner systems in use is shown in Fig. 3.3.

All breathing systems have
    an input of fresh gas,
    a reservoir, and
    an exit for expired and excess gas.

The *input* of fresh gas usually comes through flow meters but air may be entrained if the gas supply is insufficient. The flow of gas in most systems is continuous but, in certain anaesthetic machines, gas flow commences as a result of a demand by the patient and it is therefore intermittent. This demand is signalled by a subatmospheric pressure generated in the breathing system by the patient's effort of inspiration.

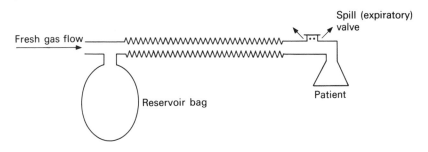

Fig.3.3. The Magill system.

The *reservoir* from which the patient breathes the prescribed mixture (or a mixture whose concentration is known approximately) is usually a bag but may be a length of gas tubing (T-piece).

The *exit* is often a spring-loaded expiratory valve but may be an open-ended tube or bag.

The reservoir bag

The name of the bag describes its main function. It is a reservoir from which the patient may breathe at his desired inspiratory flow rate. A worked example makes the point clear.

> Suppose that a patient breathes with a respiratory frequency of 20/min.
> Then, each respiratory cycle lasts 3 sec.
> If inspiration occupies ⅓ of the total time available, (I:E, 1:2)
> Then inspiration lasts 1 sec.
> If the tidal volume (volume of each breath) is 500 ml, then there is 1 sec in which the 500 ml has to reach the lungs,
> 500 ml in 1 sec,
> = 30 000 ml/min,
> = 30 litres/min.

The fresh gas flow rate normally prescribed by anaesthetists varies in different circumstances between 4 and 10 litres/min. It is clear from the above example that a reservoir is required from which gas can be drawn at an adequate rate to supply the requirements of the inspiratory flow rate. The need for an occasional deep breath can also be met.

There are other functions of the reservoir which should be noted.

Manual ventilation can readily be performed using a reservoir bag.

Monitoring of ventilation by the observation of the movements of the reservoir bag is common and good practice (see Chapter 5).

Mixing of fresh gas occurs with some of the exhaled gases, at least until the pressure within the whole system, including the bag, causes the expiratory valve to open at about 0.2 kPa (3 cmH$_2$O).

It tends to *minimize* the effect of any leak in the system and ensures the patient receives the *mixture* as prescribed.

The capacity of the bag, about 2 litres, allows a *maximal* deep breath to be taken if required.

The bag *mops* up excess pressure should obstruction develop distal to it. The inherent elasticity of the bag can accommodate many litres of gas and the pressure within it is not much greater than atmospheric until this volume is exceeded.

The bag is thus the final safety feature which protects the patient. (Normal lungs are commonly exposed to inflation pressure of 2.0-4.0 kPa (30-40 cmH$_2$O); pulmonary barotrauma may however occur in abnormal lungs at these pressures).

Elimination of carbon dioxide

This is an important function of any breathing system and it is achieved by the use of one of three methods:

a non-rebreathing system,

excessive fresh gas input,

carbon dioxide absorption.

A non-breathing or non-return system employs a valve which causes all expired gas to be discharged from the system as soon as it leaves the patient. The valve must have a low resistance and a small dead space in order for it to be efficient. The total minute volume of the patient is the same as that indicated by the flow meters, provided that the reservoir bag neither collapses nor becomes progressively more distended. The former indicates that the fresh gas flow is inadequate, and the latter that it is too great for the requirements of the patient.

The use of an excessive fresh gas input is an effective, but extravagant, way to flush the system of expired carbon dioxide. When the patient is breathing spontaneously, two to three times the minute volume as fresh gas is required (in some systems) in order to eliminate all rebreathing of carbon dioxide. Some systems are much more economical of fresh gas during controlled ventilation than others and much less fresh gas is needed. When rebreathing is allowed, but not so much as to cause the patient's arterial carbon dioxide to increase, such systems function efficiently when the fresh gas flow is as little as the patient's alveolar ventilation.

Carbon dioxide absorption is by soda lime which is contained in large, low-resistance, canisters. Soda lime is a mixture of calcium hydroxide (90%) with small amounts of sodium and potassium hydroxides. The canisters are placed in the expiratory limb of the breathing system and can be part of a circle system. Expired gases are rebreathed after they have been cleared of carbon dioxide. The arrangements of the sites for the input of fresh gas, the expiratory (dump) valve, unidirectional valves and the canisters is critical since if their relationships are inappropriate the patient may preferentially rebreathe expired gas containing carbon dioxide while the fresh gas may be dumped.

Theoretically it is possible to supply an absorption system, called in this case a closed system, with only the basal flow of oxygen, 250–300 ml/min, to meet metabolic requirements, provided that the system is leak-free. In practice the latter is difficult to achieve.

Pollution control

Interest in minimizing the fresh gas input to a breathing system has been aroused by concern about the possibly harmful effects of anaesthetic gases and vapours upon people close to patients under, or recovering from, general anaesthesia. Approaches to this problem include adsorption of the anaesthetic gases, diversion of all expired gases outside the building or the avoidance of all inhaled drugs (total intravenous anaesthesia or regional or local anaesthesia). Supplementary systems must not interfere with the proper function of breathing systems applied to patients and, in particular, must allow expiration to be passive through low-resistance expiratory valves which usually open at 0.3 kPa (3 cmH$_2$O).

Automatic ventilators

These are designed to ventilate the lungs of patients unable to breathe spontaneously, in as harmless a manner as possible.

Each ventilator has its own particular functional specification but their common purpose is to achieve an appropriate prescription, and delivery, of a minute volume of ventilation. There are some very simple machines and some which are complicated, probably to an unnecessary and expensive extent.

Many combinations of controls are offered; usually it is possible to vary the tidal volume and frequency at will. Rates of gas-flow into and out of the lungs, and the proportion of time allowed for each phase of ventilation, may often also be adjustable. Expiration can be directly to the atmosphere, against a raised pressure or assisted by a lowered (subatmospheric) pressure. Arrangements may be made to allow minimum mandatory ventilation to be administered intermittently by the machine at a slow frequency whilst the patient is spontaneously breathing during the periods in between. Variations in the concentrations of gases which may be warmed, moistened and bacteria-free can all be provided. A number of different malfunction alarms may also be found including both overpressure and disconnection alarms.

Most ventilators have a manometer incorporated in the design to display the pressure at the mouth. This pressure is that required to achieve the volume of inspiration which has been prescribed, or alternatively is the pressure which has been set so that, given no change in the patient's lung characteristics (compliance and airway resistance), the desired volume of inspiration will result. If sufficient time were allowed this mouth pressure would come to equal that in the alveoli, but inspiration is terminated before this can occur (Fig. 3.4). Sudden or steadily progressive increases in this airway pressure, or decreases in the volume of ventilation which it achieves, are important warning signs. The differential diagnosis includes obstruction to the airway, despite a tracheal tube or tracheostomy, because of the accumulation of secretions or because the tube has become kinked. A similar effect is seen when muscle tone returns to the abdominal muscles after paralysis.

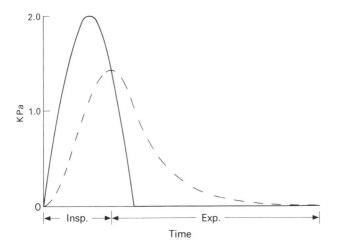

Fig. 3.4. Relationship between the pressure at the mouth and the pressure in the alveoli during the inspiratory and expiratory phases of controlled ventilation.——, Pressure at the mouth; ----, pressure in the alveoli. From Mushin W. W., Rendell-Baker L., Thompson P. W. & Mapleson W. W. (1980) *Automatic Ventilation of the Lungs*, 3rd Edn, Blackwell Scientific Publications, Oxford, with permission.

A sudden or progressive decline in the mouth pressure indicates that there is a leak in the system. This is frequently the result of disconnection of the patient from the ventilator or a failure of the cuff of the tracheal tube to make an effective seal.

It is important to understand that most, but not all, of the pressure at the mouth is transmitted into the chest. Fig. 3.4 shows this relationship. The effects of this raised airway pressure are described in Chapter 7.

Spirometers for the measurement of the volume of ventilation are either attached to the expiratory port or incorporated within the ventilator.

Oxygen therapy

This is the application of the principles of breathing systems to which reference has already been made. Oxygen is no less of a drug than any other merely because it is present in the atmosphere and, in the proper concentrations, is essential to life. (Both carbon dioxide and nitrous oxide are present in the atmosphere in minute concentrations but no one would deny they are drugs.)

Oxygen is dangerous if it is administered in high concentrations for anything other than brief periods. It is less dangerous if the concentration is restricted to about 40%, which is probably harmless no matter how long it is breathed. It should be understood, however, that notwithstanding the real risks of oxygen therapy, hypoxia is life-threatening and oxygen should never be withheld if a life is endangered by its lack. Hence it is important to know, by measurement, the concentrations of oxygen which are to be breathed by patients. (It is not certain whether oxygen *causes* retrolental fibroplasia, bronchoplastic dysplasia or the adult respiratory distress syndrome but these conditions are associated with high concentrations of oxygen.)

Oxygen analysis

Later in this book the importance of accurate knowledge of oxygen concentration is emphasised repeatedly. There are several types of oxygen analyser which can be used for static samples. Breath-by-breath analysis is not commonly required but mass spectrometers can be employed for this purpose. The fact that oxygen is strongly attracted to a magnetic field (paramagnetic) is utilized in some analysers; the movement of oxygen through an electrolyte is exploited in fuel cell analysers; and dry polarographic electrodes are also used.

Oxygen and air-mixing devices are based either on separate flow meters for each gas or on air entrainment by an oxygen-driven injector. Fig. 3.5 illustrates the principle upon which several familiar devices depend (portable suction apparatus and high air flow oxygen enrichment masks). The acceleration of gas through the orifice results in a region of reduced lateral pressure just beyond the jet. This reduction in pressure causes gas to be drawn through the ports and entrained into the diffuser tube. Provided that there is no back pressure, the proportions of driving and entrained gas remain fixed and are determined solely by the driving flow and the diameter of the jet.

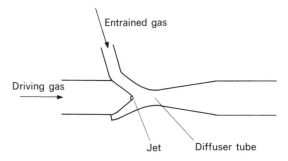

Fig. 3.5. The principle of an injector.

When air and oxygen are delivered from separate flow meters rough calculation of the inspired oxygen is simple:

2 litres/min oxygen
plus
2 litres/min air $\left(\text{i.e. } \dfrac{20}{100} \times 2 = 0.4 \text{ l/min oxygen}\right)$

Therefore, the final concentration $\left(\dfrac{2.4}{4.0} \times 100\right)$ is 60%.

Uncontrolled oxygen therapy

Simple masks are used for postoperative patients. Provided that the inspired concentration of oxygen is not at all critical this is acceptable practice. The MC mask (Mary Catterall) which has no reservoir (see Fig. 3.6) is a common example. The absence of a reservoir and the fact

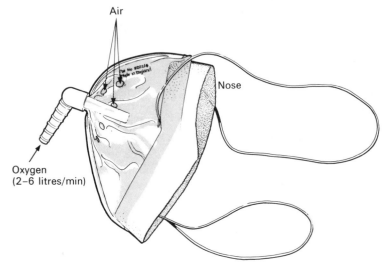

Fig. 3.6.　The Mary Catterall mask.

that wall-mounted flow meters cannot deliver more than 10–15 litres/
min of oxygen ensure that the patient cannot receive more than about
35% oxygen during normal ventilation. This concentration may vary
widely according to the patient's ventilation. If hypoventilation occurs
the inspired oxygen increases and vice versa. There can be no certainty
about the inspired oxygen concentration and therefore this mask should
be neither used for controlled oxygen therapy nor should interpretation
of arterial blood gas tensions be attempted when this mask is in use.
Similar restrictions on use exist for all masks, speculae, or cannulae
which do not have a reservoir.

Controlled oxygen therapy

This is particularly required for patients with respiratory inadequacy,
who are breathing spontaneously but whose respiratory drive may be
provided by hypoxaemia rather than the normal stimulus from carbon
dioxide. Such patients already have hypercapnia and theoretically the
administration of high concentrations of oxygen might cause apnoea.
Thus therapy with limited (controlled) oxygen is indicated. Venturi
masks (high air flow oxygen enrichment masks) work on the injector
principle and the concentration of oxygen which they provide, when

used according to the instructions, varies by only about within 1% of that specified. Fig. 3.7 shows the device. The flow rate downstream from the jet, in the absence of back pressure, is of the order of 50 litres/ min. This is in excess of the normal inspiratory flow rate: no physical reservoir is therefore required to ensure that the patient receives the prescribed mixture irrespective of the level of ventilation. A wide range of oxygen concentrations is theoretically possible. However, the masks designed for higher concentrations of oxygen have different entrainment ratios, do not produce such high total flow rates and so are probably less reliable than those designed for lower oxygen concentrations.

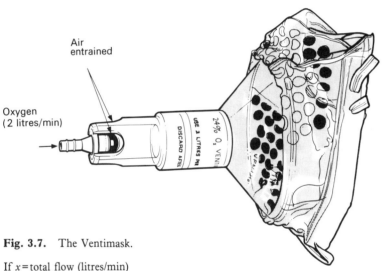

Fig. 3.7. The Ventimask.

If x = total flow (litres/min)
and 0.24 is the final concentration of oxygen
and 2 litres/min oxygen is supplied then,

$$\frac{0.21 \, (x-2)+2}{x} = 0.24$$

$$\therefore \ 0.03x = 1.58$$

$$\therefore \qquad x = 52.6$$

52.6 litres/min is in excess of the calculated inspiratory flow rate given on page 30 and is unchanged in the absence of back pressure hence, the patient breathes the inspired concentration prescribed.

Pure oxygen (i.e. 100%) is occasionally required for therapeutic purposes and it should already be clear that a reservoir bag is essential. The
BLB mask (Boothby, Lovelace and Bulbulian) is one such mask which
incorporates an expiratory valve and a reservoir bag. Pressurized pass-
enger aircraft carry similar masks for emergency use in the event of
decompression (Fig. 3.8). Another convenient apparatus is, of course,
an anaesthetic breathing system (Fig. 3.9).

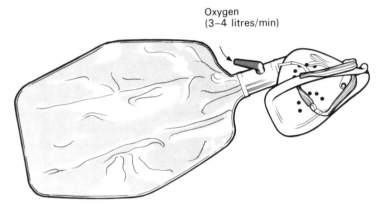

Fig. 3.8. A disposable mask with reservoir bag.

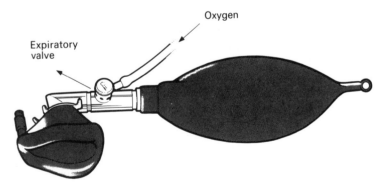

Fig. 3.9. Anaesthetic breathing system for the administration of 100% oxygen.

The occasions on which 100% oxygen may be required are summarized for convenience here (with the principle involved in brackets).

Anaesthesia (safety, protection from apnoea)
    preoxygenation – before induction of anaesthesia or electroconvulsive therapy, inflation of lungs
    – before laryngoscopy and tracheal intubation
    – before and after tracheal suction
Resuscitation (increases pressure gradient)
    during and after cardiac arrest
    florid pulmonary oedema
Measurement (eliminates effect of nitrogen gas exchange)
    assessment of arterial hypoxaemia
Miscellaneous (work them out for yourself)
    radiotherapy,
    hyperbaric medicine,
    pneumothorax,
    pneumatosis coli,
    overwhelming anaerobic infections,
    carbon monoxide poisoning.

4. Pharmacology in anaesthetics: the general anaesthetic

The course of a general anaesthetic may consist of as many as six different parts:

premedication,
induction,
maintenance,
reversal,
recovery, and
postoperative periods.

The drugs employed in each part interact with those in the others and these interactions are important. Detailed specific pharmacology for many of the drugs is not relevant to undergraduate medical students but there are examples of more general principles which are.

In addition to the above a general anaesthetic is not only a pharmacological exercise but it is also (it is to be hoped!) a balance between the action of drugs and the stimuli from surgery. Prior to, and after, a stimulus the 'pure' pharmacological effect of a drug may be seen. A patient, for example, after premedication and intravenous induction may be breathing nitrous oxide, oxygen and halothane quietly: breathing is regular, blood pressure and pulse are stable, and all the signs are that the patient is anaesthetized. This tranquil state may rapidly disappear if surgery is commenced before the tension of halothane in the brain has been raised sufficiently to prevent reaction to the stimulus: the time that this takes depends on a number of factors which will be considered later. The state of anaesthesia is achieved when the effect of the particular surgical stimulus is obtunded, but not necessarily abolished, by the action of drugs.

Drug dosage, in common with so many other biological phenomena, is subject to biological variation (Fig. 4.1). A routine, or arbitrary dose may be either excessive or inadequate for different patients in the population, whilst in a proportion the dose may achieve the desired effect. Age, sex, body weight are easily determined patient-variables whilst distribution volume, protein binding, fat solubility, ionization, metabolism and excretion are the fundamental processes about which we would like to know but cannot. (The extent to which each of these processes are active also varies from

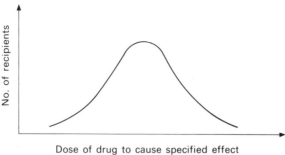

Fig. 4.1.   Curve of normal (Gaussian) distribution.

patient to patient and it is surprising that a satisfactory dose-effect relationship is ever achieved.)

The clinical practice of anaesthesia is often a compromise. Many
drugs are by custom administered in fixed dosage; minor modifications
in dosage are sometimes based on the necessarily limited number of
facts concerning the patient which are known. The effects of some other
drugs given during anaesthesia are monitored very carefully and the
dosage adjusted from minute to minute.

Premedication

There are two distinct aims in the use of premedicant drugs. One is to
prevent parasympathomimetic effects of anaesthetics and the other is
related to the need to provide relief from anxiety or pain, to provide
active sedation or to encourage amnesia: these drugs are all grouped
together for convenience as centrally-acting drugs.

Parasympatholytic drugs

Anticholinergic drugs are used to prevent *salivation* and *bronchial
secretions* in response to the stimulus of dry objects in the mouth such as
airways or tracheal tubes. (An example of a similar well-known stimulus
is the effect of a dental instrument which stimulates secretions which
need to be removed by continuous suction). Some inhaled agents are
also irritant and stimulate secretions actively, but they are almost of
historical interest only (particularly ether). Laryngeal reflexes are active
in the light planes of anaesthesia, and even small amounts of saliva can
provoke laryngeal spasm.

These drugs protect the heart against dysrhythmias particularly *bradycardia* caused by:

> concentrations of inhaled drugs (halothane, cyclopropane or trichloroethylene), which by being irritant to the respiratory tract cause reflex bradycardia,
>
> instrumentation of the airway,
>
> drugs with parasympathomimetic side effects (suxamethonium),
>
> parasympatholytic drugs also have some *antiemetic* effect, notably, hyoscine.

Centrally-acting drugs

There are several different types which may be prescribed.

Anxiolytic drugs are used to reduce the risk of dysrhythmias caused by high levels of circulating catecholamines but they should not depress the patient to an extent sufficient to cause sleep.

Sedative drugs, such as short or medium duration barbiturates, large doses of anxiolytic drugs or neuroleptic drugs are used to produce drowsiness or sleep, on the assumption that this is pleasant for the patient, but they may interfere with recovery from painful operations and cause restlessness or excitement in the postoperative period. (Neuroleptic drugs are powerful sedatives which produce dissociation from the environment. They are widely used in psychiatry: droperidol and haloperidol.)

Analgesic drugs relieve patients who are in pain at the time of operation (ischaemia, fractures, abdominal emergencies), but may cause dysphoria instead of the desired euphoria in patients who are not. The amount of general anaesthetic required subsequently is not reduced much by the premedication although the minimal alveolar concentration (page 55) of an inhaled agent is reduced. Background analgesia is also provided for the postoperative period.

Amnesic drugs. Some anxiolytics produce anterograde amnesia (that is, for the period after the drug has been administered) and they may be used deliberately for this effect. It is assumed that if an event is forgotten it has been also without lasting effect. The benzodiazepine drugs are the most common group used for this purpose. Lorazepam is long acting but temazepam is much more brief in its action.

Antiemetic drugs are essential when potent narcotic analgesics are employed in premedication (or subsequently during the anaesthetic itself). These often interact with other drugs, particularly the sedatives, and increase the degree of somnolence which results. Nausea, retching or vomiting can often be prevented and an attempt should always be made to do so. The phenothiazine drugs and droperidol are popular for this purpose.

The specific pharmacology of each and every drug used in preparing patients for anaesthesia is outside the scope of this book. The practice of anaesthetists frequently changes and the number of available drugs increases, so no scheme of 'standard' drug premedication is provided. *Every patient needs an individual prescription.*

Factors important in determining drug dosage

Preoperative discussion

Drugs are less important than a full, frank and friendly description of the whole process. Humanitarian consideration is essential and the anaesthetist who omits this is hardly worthy of his courtesy title of doctor. The reinforcement effect of this explanation on the subsequent effect of a drug, if one is given, the *placebo effect*, is an important additional benefit. Many patients do not, however, want to receive drugs with prolonged effect once they have had a proper explanation of the proposed procedure.

There is little opportunity to improve on its effects after a premedicant has been given. In other parts of anaesthetic practice dosage of drugs can often be adjusted until a desired effect is achieved. The degree of patient satisfaction which is attained preoperatively depends on how critically that effect is analysed. Hence new drugs are often enthusiastically acclaimed by their protagonists; subsequent evaluation often fails to confirm these initial impressions. (This occurrence is frequent throughout therapeutics but is nowhere more common than in the practice of drug premedication.)

Body weight is an important variable: the grossly obese patient may not require a sedative or an analgesic drug to be given per kilogram body weight, but in proportion to the degree of anxiety or pain which is experienced; husky rugby players, even medical students, are often much more apprehensive prior to surgery than one would otherwise anticipate. There are racial and even geographical differences in degrees of preoperative anxiety which must also be considered.

It is clear that body size, and thus body weight, may indicate racial background or nutrition, and these may affect dilution, metabolism or protein binding. In general, while the extremes of body weight influence drug dosage of premedicants small variations do not.

Age, in general, is less important than body weight as a determinant of drug dosage. In children it is naive, not to say dangerous, to base dosage on age since disasters resulting from overdosage have occurred. The elderly often seem more tranquil and resigned and do not require large doses of anxiolytic drugs; if the dosages given are weight-adjusted the elderly are not particularly sensitive to sedatives or analgesics. Atropine is usually substituted for hyoscine since it is claimed that the latter causes excitement or delirium in elderly patients.

Intercurrent disease, even the surgical diagnosis, may determine the choice of premedicant drugs. Oral drugs cannot be used if the patient cannot swallow or if there is persistent vomiting.

Intercurrent therapy and drug history (including abuse). Long-term therapy with anxiolytics or sedatives may result in habituation, with the result that the patient is so used to their effects that larger doses than anticipated are required. Metabolism may also be altered. This mechanism may, for example, be responsible for prolonged unconsciousness after anaesthesia. Monoamine oxidase inhibitors interact with narcotics (see Chapter 2).

Alcohol intake. The effect of this can be compared with the intended effect of premedicant drugs. The patient's sensitivity to alcohol is also a useful guide to the likely response to sedative or similar drugs.

Routes of administration of premedicant drugs (Fig. 4.2)

Oral drugs are preferred by many patients who, not unnaturally, may dislike injections. Absorption may be unreliable and is certainly variable. Larger doses tend therefore to be used but these carry the risk that *all* the dose may on occasion be absorbed. Oral analgesics are significantly less efficacious but many anxiolytics, sedatives or amnesic drugs are given satisfactorily by this route.

Subcutaneous injection is less commonly used nowadays because absorption is unreliable.

Intramuscular injection is usually associated with better absorption but the needle injection is painful, the drug itself may cause pain, and its action may be prolonged to an unwanted extent. An anomalous effect is found with diazepam which is less well absorbed following intramuscular injection than following oral administration; injection also causes pain.

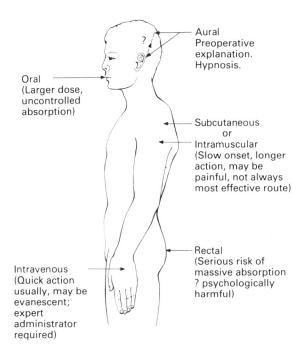

Fig. 4.2. Routes of administration of preoperative preparation.

Intravenous premedication is usually reserved for emergencies. The effect is rapid in onset but short acting, and usually requires medical administration.

Rectal administration also carries the risk of massive unexpected absorption and patients must be observed continuously after injection. Thiopentone and other drugs have been used, particularly in children, by this route.

Induction

This is the second part of an anaesthetic. It may, in the unpremedicated patient, be the only part of the procedure which is remembered subsequently but many patients who have received premedication totally forget induction. The *aim* is not to anaesthetize but merely to start that process quickly and pleasantly: it is defined here as the induction of

sleep by chemical hypnosis. Psychological hypnosis is used by a few
doctors to achieve induction, particularly in children, but this is usually
followed by conventional drugs.

There are four practical routes by which anaesthetic drugs may be
introduced into the body. These are:

    intravenous,
    rectal,
    intramuscular,
    inhalation.

Intravenous induction agents are ideally ones which have:

    rapid onset,
    profound effect,
    brief duration,
    no interactions,
    wide therapeutic indices.

The barbiturates

Many of the barbiturate series of drugs have been used in the past and
a few still are, notably methohexitone (a methylated oxybarbiturate),
but the *thio*barbiturates are much the most important group. These
compounds have a sulphur atom substituted in barbituric acid. They
are presented as water-soluble sodium salts for parenteral use and their
action begins within one arm-brain circulation time. The example of
this group of world-wide importance is thiopentone sodium. In keeping
with the philosophy of this book the detailed pharmacology and clinical
use of these drugs will not be described but a few important points must
be made.

Pharmacokinetics

More experiments have been performed with thiopentone than with
any other intravenous induction agent and so much of what follows is
based on these findings. It is widely assumed that the observations on
thiopentone are applicable to other intravenous barbiturate drugs.

Comparisons between intravenous induction agents are not simple
because, by definition, the effects are temporary and thus are constantly
changing. In contrast to the inhaled anaesthetics, equilibrium concen-

trations are never reached after small doses, and larger doses may produce acute tolerance or very prolonged effects.

Comparisons of 'potency' between drugs are not very informative. The concept of therapeutic index (the ratio of the therapeutic dose to that which produces undesirable effects) is also unhelpful in relation to use of anaesthetic drugs since, apart from extremes, a particular effect may not be undesirable in a particular clinical circumstance. Finally, many dosage problems in anaesthetics are solved by reference to the axiom 'enough, for a given effect, is the correct amount'. Methohexitone is generally stated to be three times as potent, milligram for milligram, as thiopentone.

Protein binding

This accounts for about 65% of an injected dose of thiopentone; albumin is the main site. The bound fraction cannot take part in any action on the central nervous system since this depends upon diffusion, and proteins of the molecular size of albumin do not cross the blood-brain barrier.

Reduced amounts of thiopentone are required in patients with absolutely or relatively low plasma protein levels; for example, in liver disease, hypovolaemia or undernutrition. Sulphafurazole interferes with the binding of thiopentone, and has been shown experimentally to reduce significantly the dose required for a specific effect.

Ionization

Access to brain tissue is correlated with the fat solubility of that part of the molecule which is un-ionized at physiological concentrations of hydrogen ion. This is 60% for thiopentone and 75% for methohexitone. The un-ionized fraction is highly soluble in fat, thus thiopentone is both quickly effective in the brain, and can be quickly removed from the brain by the process of diffusion. The difference in the degree of ionization of thiopentone and methohexitone may account for the greater potency and quicker recovery associated with the latter drug.

The degree of ionization of a drug is expressed in relation to the hydrogen ion activity (pH), and the point on the pH scale at which a drug is 50% ionized is called the dissociation constant (pK). For thiopentone this is 7.6, whereas for methohexitone it is 7.9.

Distribution

Tissue uptake is determined by blood flow and uptake occurs almost simultaneously with the brain in the liver and kidney, and later in muscle. Notwithstanding the high fat solubility of thiopentone, the limiting factor is the blood flow which prevents the rapid and immediate loss from the circulation into fat, because this is poorly supplied with blood. Muscle uptake is, however, extensive, and muscle is an early recipient of injected drugs. Later, when the brain level has fallen below that which causes hypnosis, the level in fat tissue rises, so that approximately one-third of the dose of thiopentone is found in fat by about 90 minutes after injection.

Distribution of drugs in different tissues is compared by means of partition coefficients, which relate the amounts present at equilibrium in the two phases under consideration. Fat solubility is similar to solubility in certain oils, and oil/water partition coefficients are, for example, often used for comparative purposes. Thiopentone is 1.36 times more soluble than methohexitone in fat. Thus a smaller proportion of a dose of thiopentone is immediately available for metabolism in the liver.

Metabolism

Metabolism in the liver is important in the early reduction of plasma concentrations and, later, in the detoxification of thiopentone. Loss of liver function has to be extreme before clinical effects are obvious. The kidneys excrete the products of metabolism eventually but only a very small part of the unaltered drug is found in the urine since the un-ionized portion is rapidly reabsorbed.

The placenta offers no barrier to thiopentone and the fetus is brought rapidly into equilibrium with the maternal thiopentone level.

Dose-dependent phenomena

Repeated doses of thiopentone can cause the brain to reach an equilibrium with the level in the arterial blood supplying it and, since the remainder of the tissues in the body also have increased drug levels, uptake in these tissues ceases to be an effective means of ensuring brevity of action. Thus subsequent increments of thiopentone need to be much smaller.

In contrast to the inhaled drugs, recovery from thiopentone anaesthesia occurs irrespective of the plasma levels of the drug. Fig. 4.3 shows that the plasma level of thiopentone at the moment of awakening increases with increasing dose of thiopentone: if plasma level were *the* determinant of awakening there would be a flat relationship at some plasma level; there is not.

Whereas with many other drugs a large loading dose is used therapeutically, with thiopentone the reverse seems to be desirable. 'Acute tolerance' is a phenomenon which is not explicable satisfactorily and which is shown by thiopentone. If a large dose is given initially, subsequent doses must also be large to achieve the same effect; rapid administration also seems to have the same effect.

Sensitivity

Synergism between other barbiturates, phenothiazines, benzodiazepines, opiates and thiopentone occurs commonly and is useful, provided that it is foreseen. If a patient is tolerant to other sedatives cross tolerance to thiopentone occurs. Anaphylaxis is a small but real risk.

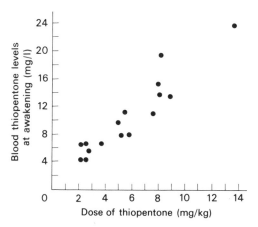

Fig. 4.3. The dependence of blood thiopentone level at awakening on the dose of thiopentone. From Dundee J. W., Price H. L., & Dripps, R. D. (1956). Acute tolerance to thiopentone in man. *Br. J. Anaesthesia* **28,** 344, with permission.

Important rarities

Thiopentone as its sodium salt in solution is very alkaline (pH about 10.8) and is very irritant to tissues if injected outside a vein. *Intra-arterial injection* is a serious matter: arterial blockage from precipitation of thiopentone crystals, arterial spasm from noradrenaline release, and arteritis with subsequent arterial thrombosis all combine to cause, in the worst cases, gangrene. Immediate treatment consists of a variety of manoeuvres designed to increase blood flow to the affected area as a result of vasodilatation. Finger, hand or even limb amputation may be required at a much later stage. The use of dilute solutions of thiopentone at injection sites distant from arteries has reduced the frequency of this accident to that of a rarity.

Porphyria is an inborn error of metabolism of porphyrin: *acute intermittent porphyria* is one of several diseases in the group found more commonly in Scandinavia and South Africa than elsewhere. Demyelination of nerves is a feature of the disease and the patient may present with abdominal pain, muscle paralysis, or weakness or psychiatric symptons. If barbiturates, including thiopentone, are given the paralysis may rapidly extend and become catastrophically permanent. Amongst other drugs which may aggravate the condition are sulphonamides and some sedatives e.g. dichloralphenazone (Welldorm) and glutethimide (Doriden). An important clue to the probable aetiology of this condition is that all these drugs induce an enzyme (aminolaevulic acid synthetase) which is already present in excess of normal in patients suffering from porphyria.

Non-barbiturate intravenous induction agents

There are three groups of drugs which need consideration under this heading, each for its own reason. These are:

    neurolept anaesthetic drugs,
    rapidly metabolized drugs,
    dissociative drugs.

Some of the drugs which come into this classification are either no longer used widely or have never passed beyond the interest of the curious. Each group, however, provides examples of different pharmacological actions which are important.

Neurolepsis is a term used to describe the condition and appearance of a patient who has received a potent but specific sedative, usually a butyrophenone derivative, for example droperidol. The state combines a reluctance to move spontaneously (catatonia) with a detachment from the reality of the environment (dissociation). Useful additional properties of droperidol are that it is a very effective antiemetic (see below) and it causes some alpha-adrenergic blockade. The latter effect is claimed to improve peripheral circulation through organs as well as through skin and hypotension is a real risk in hypovolaemic patients. Large doses may cause Parkinson-like symptoms and signs of extrapyramidal stimulation. The tranquil appearance of a patient may hide feelings of extreme agitation if the drug is given by itself.

The combination of droperidol, or any other major tranquilliser, with potent analgesic drugs has become known as *neurolept anaesthesia.* The benefit of the antiemetic effect of droperidol is now obvious because these analgesics are powerful stimulants to vomiting. Increased skeletal muscle tone and apnoea develop after induction with this combination of drugs and thus muscle paralysis, intubation and controlled ventilation with nitrous oxide and oxygen are required. The process of induction is slow. Droperidol may take up to 20 minutes to reach its peak of action and its effects are also prolonged, but provided no synergistic drugs are used, initial recovery is prompt.

It is claimed, without overwhelming evidence, that this type of anaesthesia provides better protection for the whole organism against the noxious stimuli of surgery.

Dissociative anaesthesia refers to the total state of detachment and profound analgesia to stimuli of superficial pain. There is one drug only in this group, ketamine, which produces the above state about 2 minutes after intravenous injection. However, there are many disadvantages to its use: the patient may move in response to surgical stimulation, there is no muscular relaxation, salivation is excessive, arterial and intracranial hypertension occur, and unpleasant dreams, during and after surgery, are commonly recalled. These undesirable effects can be eliminated by other procedures or drugs, and it is possible that future pharmaceutical development may provide a single satisfactory drug. The arterial hypertension can be useful and some anaesthetists advocate the drug where hypotension is known to exist preoperatively and also suggest its use at the site of major disasters for primary surgery (amputation of a trapped limb).

Rapidly metabolized intravenous induction agents regularly appear on the market and equally regularly disappear from it. The potential advantage of these drugs is that their action is terminated in a predictable interval and that no residual action remains. A derivative of eugenol (propanidid) and a mixture of two steroids (Althesin) were two such drugs, both of which have been removed from the market. Propanidid is hydrolysed in the plasma under the influence of the enzyme plasma cholinesterase and Althesin is metabolized by the liver. Cumulation following repeated doses of propanidid is much less than that following thiopentone; the duration of action of Althesin is intermediate between the other two drugs and this may indicate that metabolism and redistribution account for its brief action. The result is that recovery from anaesthesia is more complete and relatively free from hangover effects than that following thiobarbiturates, although initial recovery may not be more than a few seconds quicker. The serious limitation to the use of these drugs was that they were both made soluble by Cremophor which has been blamed for the hypersensitivity reactions (cutaneous vasodilatation, bronchospasm and hypotension) which occur following injections of both of these drugs. It is, however, interesting that this substance is still used to solubilize Vitamin K and cyclosporin.

Etomidate, an imidazole derivative, is a potent water soluble intravenous anaesthetic agent which, when injected without any pretreatment, commonly causes pain in the vein and many patients show extra involuntary movements. Recovery happens rapidly and the patients are more clear-headed than after barbiturates. (Infusions were used for the provision of sedation in intensive care units but the finding that the formation of corticosteroids was suppressed led to the abandonment of their use.)

Propofol, an isopropyl phenol, now dissolved in a soya bean emulsion, is another rapidly redistributed and metabolized intravenous anaesthetic. It too is associated with prompt complete recovery and few side effects.

Midazolam is a rapidly acting benzodiazepine which produces sedation and sleep 2-3 minutes after intravenous injection. This is in marked contrast to the other intravenous anaesthetics mentioned which induce anaesthesia within one minute. Recovery is quicker than that after diazepam but slower than after thiopentone.

Critique of intravenous induction agents

The intravenous thiobarbiturates are in a superior position in relation to any new drug because they have been in continuous and world-wide use since 1934. All their successors, whether barbiturates or not, have in spite of some significant advantages, also some clear practical disadvantages which they share amongst themselves or have as unique characteristics. For example, methohexitone causes pain in the upper arm when injected intravenously at the wrist or hand. It is associated with a greater number of annoying, but not life-threatening, reflex movements than thiopentone: hiccup, pronation of the arm, and cough. The more recently introduced drugs mentioned above represent important improvements and it is possible that they, or their derivatives, will come to challenge seriously the thiobarbiturates. The method of total intravenous anaesthesia, which is in its infancy, depends on the availability of non-cumulative short acting drugs and these are now becoming available. Short acting potent narcotic and non-narcotic analgesics can be used without the addition of nitrous oxide or a volatile inhalation agent to maintain anaesthesia, and thus the problem of atmospheric pollution is avoided. Nevertheless, in terms of induction of anaesthesia, the equal of thiopentone has yet to be discovered.

Other routes for induction of anaesthesia

Rectal and intramuscular routes have been used for those patients, particularly children, who have to undergo repeated general anaesthesia, have unsuitable veins or who are psychologically disturbed.

Rectal administration of thiopentone is effective but not without serious hazard since the patient is liable to the same complications as those which follow intravenous induction. Absorption is inversely related to the amount of faecal matter present in the rectum. The effects of an injection are variable probably because of this, but also because of different rates of absorption according to the different routes of venous drainage. It is necessary to provide a high degree of skill and care following rectal thiopentone and hence, with the advent of other drugs, this method has become less appropriate.

The *intramuscular* route is only seldom used for barbiturate drugs nowadays because ketamine is, in many ways, more satisfactory. Thiopentone is less suitable than methohexitone since the latter is less irritant, but ketamine is less irritant than either. The large dose which is required may result in prolonged action and duration of any adverse reactions is also prolonged.

Inhalation induction of anaesthesia

Inhalational anaesthetic drugs can be used to commence an anaesthetic. It was, of course, the first method used historically and comparison with the intravenous method is instructive.

The aim of an inhalation induction is not the same as that of an intravenous induction. The induction period is nearly always the induction of surgical anaesthesia; once one inhalant, for example halothane, is used the same agent may be continued throughout the operation for maintenance whereas intravenous thiopentone is given solely for hypnosis. However, cyclopropane is sometimes used solely for induction in very ill patients or in children.

Inhalation induction is slower than intravenous but is more readily controlled and may therefore be safer. A test dose of an intravenous agent, once given is irretrievably inside the patient but, to some extent the effect of an inhalant can be reversed by reduction of the inspired concentration and controlled ventilation of the lungs if required.

Intravenous agents are discarded early in their pharmaceutical development if local irritation, pain or histamine release is noticed. Ether is very irritant to the respiratory tract, but it was not discarded because of this fact. The rate of increase in concentration with which it is given is gradual and induction is therefore very slow. Other more recent inhalant drugs do not have this disadvantage, although isoflurane is irritant when given to unpremedicated patients.

Intravenous and inhalation induction of anaesthesia are hazardous procedures and both are associated with the sudden life-threatening complications such as aspiration of vomit, severe dysrhythmias with haemodynamic effects or profound hypotension from peripheral vasodilatation.

Inhalation induction is used electively for those patients who have no superficial veins, who are petrified of venepuncture and by some anaesthetists for children. In emergency surgery on a moribund patient anaesthesia may be induced more safely by inhalational anaesthesia than by the intravenous agents.

Maintenance

This period follows induction and is that during which the surgical or other procedure is performed. It may appear to the uninitiated onlooker that very little happens during maintenance and, it is true that, during an uncomplicated anaesthetic, this should be the case. It is probably not the most dangerous part of an anaesthetic but from the surgical viewpoint, it is one of the most important (see Chapter 5). There are several pharmacological aspects which are worthy of consideration.

How is anaesthesia maintained?

There are several methods and many drugs from which an anaesthetist may, somewhat arbitrarily, choose. Inhaled drugs (halothane, trichloroethylene, methoxyflurane, enflurane, isoflurane) may be used as supplements to nitrous oxide. Parenteral, usually intravenous, analgesics (morphine, pethidine, fentanyl, phenoperidine, alfentanil, nalbuphine), may be used similarly. The latter method is often combined with muscle relaxation (caused by specific drugs) and the effect of this combination makes controlled ventilation of the lungs essential; the former method is more commonly applied when ventilation is to be spontaneous. Regional analgesic techniques may be occasionally combined with general anaesthesia (see Chapter 6).

Inhaled anaesthetics

Table 4.1 Minimal alveolar concentrations

Agent	Concentration %
(Cyclopropane	9.2)
(Diethyl ether	1.92)
Enflurane	1.68
Halothane	0.76
Isoflurane	1.15
(Methoxyflurane	0.16)
Nitrous oxide	101
(Trichloroethylene	0.2)

The Minimal Alveolar Concentration (MAC)

This is a concept in the study of pharmacodynamics of inhaled anaesthetic drugs equivalent to that of the familiar Effective Dose beloved by pharmacologists. It is defined as that concentration in the alveoli at equilibrium which is sufficient just to prevent reaction to a standard surgical stimulus in half the (surgical) population. It is a useful statistic by means of which comparisons between anaesthetic drugs and their effects can be made. Table 4.1 lists some values. Comparisons of specific changes in a physiological variable can be made by measuring that variable before and after exposure to MAC (and multiples of MAC) for a number of anaesthetic agents. Fig. 4.4 is an example which demonstrates this. It can be seen that for equivalent MAC values the ventilation of a group of patients varied according to the agents used. B has greater depressant action on ventilation than A. This might be due to specific pharmacological actions of B, or it might be due to the fact that A is so irritant to the respiratory tract that ventilation is stimulated, even when the patient is anaesthetized with a concentration which is three times MAC.

The use of MAC values in this way assumes that equilibrium has been achieved, that is, no further uptake of anaesthetic is occurring. Equilibrium is in terms of partial pressure and implies that the partial pressure in the alveoli is the same as that in the blood; it does not refer to the amount or concentration of anaesthetic.

A moment's reflection reveals that *complete* equilibrium between all tissues and the blood cannot occur except after a very long time

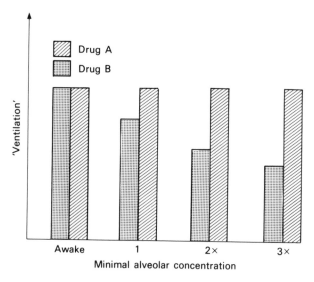

Fig. 4.4. Use of minimal alveolar concentrations of two drugs to compare their effects on ventilation (see text).

because, although most inhaled anaesthetics are very soluble in fat, this is relatively poorly supplied with blood and uptake therein continues. Equilibrium between blood and brain does not take long because the range of solubilities of anaesthetics in brain is not wide and the brain perfusion with blood is lavish. It is really this equilibrium concentration which is involved when MAC is measured.

Uptake of anaesthetic from the lung depends on:

removal by the blood flowing through the lung,

uptake and solubility of the agent in blood,

amount of agent already in the blood.

Solubilities of gases or vapours vary widely with the various agents, but it is sufficient here to state that two extreme examples – very soluble (methoxyflurane) and very insoluble (nitrous oxide) – differ considerably in their pharmacokinetics. Insoluble agents reach equilibrium between blood and gas (or tissue) very rapidly, within a few minutes, whilst soluble agents may take many hours to achieve this state.

There are several inhaled anaesthetic drugs on the market whose detailed merits are not relevant here. One drug, halothane (see page 111), although not without some disadvantages in specific circumstances, is used in about 50% of all anaesthetics. It is intermediate between nitrous oxide and methoxyflurane as far as solubility is concerned. Cyclopropane is relatively insoluble and trichloroethylene is very soluble; in addition both these drugs have specific limitations. Enflurane and isoflurane are both less soluble than halothane and this is responsible for the claims of more rapid induction with, and recovery from, anaesthesia with these agents.

When inhaled drugs are used for maintenance of anaesthesia with controlled ventilation, low inspired concentrations of supplementary drugs are used since ventilation is one of the variables of delivery of anaesthetic to the alveoli. In contrast, when spontaneous ventilation is used to deliver the anaesthetic to the alveoli, the inspired concentration is varied by the anaesthetist in response to the reaction of the patient to surgical stimulation, but the ventilation is determined by the patient. In practice, inspired concentrations during maintenance are usually about 50% greater than MAC during spontaneous ventilation, and about half MAC during controlled ventilation with muscle relaxants.

The study of pharmacokinetics of inhaled anaesthetics is a large postgraduate subject but it should now be clear that physical differences between agents, their individual pharmacological effects and pre-existing physiological function all interact in a complex manner. Additive effects are found when more than one inhaled agent is administered at the same time; this affects both rate of uptake and MAC values (Fig. 4.5).

Analgesics

The general pharmacological principles of dissociation, protein binding and lipid solubility, which have been illustrated by reference to thiopentone, apply also to any drug administered parenterally and examples are not repeated here.

Most analgesics, which are available in a formulation compatible with parenteral administration, have been used to provide analgesia during surgical anaesthesia. Derivatives of morphine used in premedication do not have a marked effect on MAC (Fig. 4.5), but may have significant effects on the response to deeper painful stimuli. Small amounts of analgesics are used in increments to obtund the recognized signs which

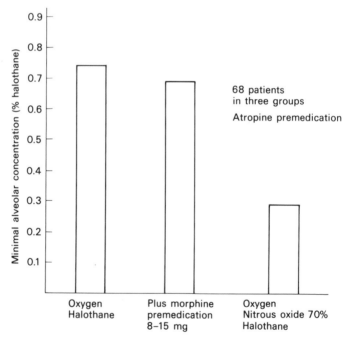

Fig. 4.5. Minimal alveolar concentrations of halothane, with morphine premedication, and with 70% nitrous oxide.

develop in response to surgical stimuli: lacrimation, pupillary dilatation, sweating, hypertension, tachycardia. The doses required to achieve this vary widely in an unpredictable manner, but dosage is kept to the minimum required.

Each drug used has other effects than those on reactions to painful stimuli. Hypotension, due either to peripheral vasodilatation or to a direct effect on myocardial contractility, is the commonest. The actions of sedatives, hypnotics or tranquillizers are increased if analgesics are administered concomitantly. This may be due to true synergism or because, in the absence of pain produced by the analgesic, the sedative has no stimulus to foreshorten or modify its action.

Most, if not quite all, effective analgesics are narcotics and capable of abuse. There are therefore statutory rules of prescription and distribution which have to be followed as much by anaesthetists as by anyone else.

The subject of receptors for opiate and opioid drugs and their antagonists is a very complex one. It is sufficient to note that pure agonist drugs (fentanyl, alfentanil) cause respiratory depression which can be reversed, not only by pure antagonists (naloxone), but also by drugs which are not only analgesics but also *both* agonist and antagonist in their action (pentazocine, buprenorphine and nalbuphine). The latter series of drugs is constantly expanding.

Many narcotic analgesics also cause vomiting and although narcotic-induced vomiting does not occur during maintenance of anaesthesia but during and after recovery, it is routinely prevented by antiemetic drugs given at the same time.

Muscle relaxants

It is customary to describe two distinct types of muscle relaxant drugs, *depolarizing* and *non-depolarizing*. Both act at the neuromuscular junction. Suxamethonium effectively depolarizes the end-plate in a manner similar to acetylcholine, but for a more prolonged period and to a more profound extent. It is the most important of the group of depolarizing relaxants. Non-depolarizing relaxants prevent the action of acetylcholine and deny it access to the end-plate. About three-quarters of all general anaesthetics administered today include the use of one or more relaxants.

Suxamethonium is used for the brief profound relaxation such as required for intubation of the trachea or as part of the modification of electroconvulsive therapy. The drug is promptly hydrolysed by plasma cholinesterase and its action is usually terminated within 3–5 minutes. The fasciculation which always marks the commencement of the action of the drug results, nearly always, in the development of muscle pains on the following day. These pains can be quite severe and may easily be mistaken for a more serious condition. They are worse in patients who have had relatively trivial surgery and who are therefore mobile early in the postoperative period; the muscles of the abdomen, back, shoulders and calves are commonly affected. They subside in 24–36 hours following rest. Some anaesthetists attempt to prevent their occurrence by the use of a minute amount of a non-depolarizing relaxant prior to suxamethonium.

Non-depolarizing relaxants (tubocurarine, alcuronium, pancuronium, vecuronium, atracurium) are longer acting than is suxamethonium. They may be used by themselves for tracheal intubation and for maintenance or merely used after intubation of the trachea has been achieved with the aid of suxamethonium. Their effects are dose-dependent, but the muscles of respiration are affected to the same extent as any muscle and thus controlled ventilation is essential.

Anaesthetists are careful to distinguish between reflex response to pain and movement due to inadequate muscle paralysis: different treatment is required.

Recovery

This period can be divided into three parts:
    reversal,
    early recovery,
    late recovery.

Reversal

This part of recovery is usually very short, but it is both very important and very hazardous. It is the first part of recovery and is accomplished under the direct personal supervision of the anaesthetist and usually is conducted in the operating room.

The concentration of inhalants, other than nitrous oxide, are reduced towards the end of an anaesthetic. Estimates are made of the duration of the remainder of the operation and the inhaled concentration is reduced to zero in relation to its solubility. (A very soluble agent can be terminated earlier than an insoluble one since the brain level of the former is itself only reduced slowly.)

When spontaneous respiration has been maintained and the inspired concentration of inhalant has been reduced to zero the nitrous oxide can also be discontinued. A few moments later the patient responds to all stimuli, and therefore this last manoeuvre should not be started until surgery is over. Oxygen is given for a few minutes, otherwise nitrous oxide, which diffuses *from* the blood into the alveoli, would reduce the alveolar oxygen concentration and arterial hypoxaemia might occur.

When non-depolarizing relaxants have been used, reversal of their action is essential; even though spontaneous ventilation would almost invariably recommence, it would probably be inadequate. This reversal is usually achieved by an anticholinesterase, neostigmine or edrophonium, and is preceded by atropine to avoid the unwanted muscarinic effects (salivation, bronchial secretions, bradycardia).

If, when spontaneous ventilation returns, the respiratory rate is slow (say less than 6-8/min) a narcotic antagonist is used. Narcotic antagonists are antagonists to *all* the effects of narcotics, including analgesia, and some (nalorphine and levallorphan) even have narcotic properties themselves. One antagonist (naloxone) has no such effect and can therefore be given as a therapeutic test in cases of doubt. It is important to remember that pain relief may only be achieved with considerable difficulty after one of these drugs and large doses of analgesic may then be required. Thus, narcotic antagonists are used in the small doses which show themselves to be sufficient for the purpose intended.

Hypocapnia may contribute to the persistence of apnoea after intermittent positive pressure ventilation, but it is seldom, if ever, the sole cause. Resumption of spontaneous ventilation may be caused in hypocapnic patients merely by movement of the tracheal tube. Carbon dioxide inhalation has the effect not only of increasing the arterial tension of carbon dioxide, but also of causing a general increase in neuronal activity in the hindbrain which affects the arousal mechanism of the reticular activating system.

When spontaneous ventilation is judged to be adequate, or better, when it is measured, extubation of the trachea can be carried out. This is done when the protective laryngeal reflexes have returned and after removal of pharyngeal secretions by suction. The patient receives oxygen throughout extubation and is placed in the left lateral position.

Early recovery

This part of the recovery period is supervised somewhat distantly by the anaesthetist but directly by qualified nurses. The anaesthetist can easily be summoned if assistance is required. Oxygen therapy is continued, (see Chapter 7), observations are made on the state of unconsciousness (see Chapter 5) and analgesic drugs are administered. Antiemetic drugs (metoclopramide, cyclizine, perphenazine, droperidol) may be required. The early recovery lasts until the patient is well-oriented in time and space, and is able to protect his own airway. This usually takes no more than an hour; its duration partly depends on the duration of the anaesthetic which preceded it. Crudely this is sometimes called the 'wake-up time'. Many patients, however, fall back to sleep and have no memory of their early awakening.

Analgesia is provided in the recovery room according to patient need and as judged by the nurses (see below).

Late recovery

This is merely the continuance of the process which began as soon as anaesthetic drugs were reversed; it is the period of recovery from the anaesthetic which occurs in the ward remote from the anaesthetist. Most patients are fully recovered in a few hours after the operation. Some hangover effect may remain such as headache, dizziness and inability to concentrate.

Postoperative care

There are several particular aspects of this period of normal recovery after an operation which involve anaesthetists. Firstly, early postoperative complications may be forecast on the basis of events which have happened during the operation (for example, dysrhythmias, drug response or haemorrhage). Secondly, the surgical members of the team need to be warned of anticipated intravenous fluid requirements and alerted to the problems of sensitivity, incompatibility of additives or the risks of fluid overload which may have been encountered during the operation. Thirdly, anaesthetists are in a position to communicate their assessment of the patient's response to analgesics and their future analgesic requirements. Some anaesthetists prescribe postoperative analgesics for 24 hours themselves; others guide house staff in their prescriptions. Whichever method is used, it is likely that narcotic analgesics will not be required for longer than 24-48 hours postoperatively, when they may be replaced by milder, often orally administered, drugs.

Management of postoperative pain

The best method to determine an individual's requirements is by means of an experiment. Repeated small boluses of analgesic are given intravenously at suitable time intervals until the *patient* says that the pain has gone. This is the common practice in recovery rooms. If one to two doses of morphine are given in this manner and the patient observed continuously by trained nurses and by a doctor, an informed estimate of the effective intramuscular dose can be made. Once the pain has been relieved successfully, it is common for the relief to last 2 or more hours and then an intramuscular regimen (based on the total intravenous dose) every 4 hours may be substituted. It is important to ensure that patients actually receive the prescribed drugs and are not left in pain. The real dangers of narcotic-induced respiratory depression have probably been exaggerated in the past to the detriment of patient comfort.

This method has been further developed so that a predetermined dose of drug is delivered automatically to the patient in response to demand. A syringe pump, connected to an intravenous infusion, is controlled by a mechanism to limit the frequency of dosing and there is a simple test device to ensure that the patient does not merely press the demand button at random. Investigations using this apparatus have indicated how widely patients differ in their analgesic requirements, for example, in one group of postoperative patients after the same operation, the demands ranged between 400 and 1400 mg pethidine in one 24-hour period. Self-administration is appreciated by patients and nurses alike. There are several variations of this method with varying degrees of complexity, including the continuous infusion of narcotics. A few of these methods are somewhat hazardous and will only be found in high-dependency units.

Epidural anaesthesia can be extended to the postoperative period merely by use of an indwelling catheter (see page 107). Hypotension from overdose or unexpected spread of the solution are two hazards of uncontrolled administration, and it is probably preferable for additional doses of drugs to be supervised directly by doctors. Hypotension is treated with infusion of fluids and, rarely, with vasopressors.

The hazards of sympathetic paralysis which causes hypotension are avoided when *narcotics* are injected by the intrathecal or epidural route. Narcotic analgesics act on opiate receptors; these receptors are found in the substantia gelatinosum of the spinal cord. Preservative-free narcotics reach these areas after direct injection and cause long-lasting analgesia in the areas supplied by the segments affected. Very small amounts are required; hypotension does not occur since the sympathetic system is not affected, but respiratory depression may develop even hours after the injection. This can be reversed by naloxone. Circumoral itching occurs after spinal narcotics; nausea and vomiting may also be troublesome.

Theories of general anaesthetic action

There is no one theory to account for all drugs which *can* be anaesthetic. Gases of one atom (xenon), simple gases (nitrous oxide) and vapours (ethers) or the large molecular structures of steroids (Althesin) can all cause reversible depression of the central nervous system. Some anaesthetic drugs can also stimulate the central nervous system (or at least appear to) while at the same time apparently acting as anaesthetics (methohexitone, Althesin, ketamine, enflurane).

On the one hand, therefore, there may be several different mechanisms to explain anaesthesia and indeed there are numerous phenomena of which account needs to be taken. On the other hand, however, there are only a few sites where the neurophysiology of nerve and nerve cell can be influenced. Hence there is a paradox which is, as yet, not fully resolved, but it is more and more likely that different anaesthetic agents produce their effect by different mechanisms.

An action on the cell membrane which involves alteration in the mobility of phospholipid molecules seems a possibility. This might stretch, or even partially disrupt, the double layer of lipid in the cell membrane. The correlations of various physicochemical properties, such as oil or fat solubility, with anaesthetic potency indicate the importance of fats in the cell membranes. There is, however, now sufficient evidence to show that the action of anaesthetics is to change cell membrane proteins so that their function is altered. These proteins are held in a framework of lipids so that lipid solubility is an important feature of anaesthetic action, hence the correlation between potency and oil/water solubility.

If the phospholipids are affected first it is possible that proteins, which control ionic flux, within nervous tissue, are affected secondarily. Movement of sodium ions against an electrochemical gradient is by means of active transport and this is inhibited by many anaesthetics. This action is achieved by enzyme depression in some cases, or by reduction in oxidative metabolism in others. The increase in permeability of cell membranes to potassium ions results in an increase in the threshold of excitability of some nerve cells. Changes in membrane permeability can be shown to occur as a result of exposure to anaesthetics.

Some of the evidence quoted above is based on neurophysiological research using very atypical *in vitro* preparations which may not be precise models for drug action in the central nervous system of humans.

The application of very high pressures to model systems under the influence of anaesthetic agents reverses that anaesthetic action. Any theory which is to account for anaesthetic action must include this phenomenon, which has been demonstrated for many agents in several models, including nerve conduction but excluding synaptic transmission.

The complexity of the organization of the central nervous system is such that many different sites of action within the brain are possible. Anaesthetics act at synapses throughout the central nervous system - particularly in the brain stem, thalamus and cortex. They depress excitatory activity, and may depress or stimulate inhibitory activity. In contrast to an earlier theory, the reticular activating system is not the primary site of action of all anaesthetics. There is a general reduction of cerebral metabolic rate, but this reduction is different in different areas of the brain and also varies with the agent studied. Since the cortex is the region of the brain so obviously concerned with consciousness it is likely also to be the area which is affected by anaesthetic agents.

5. Coma and monitoring

Coma is the state of being unconscious, and there are three general types:

physiological,
pharmacological, or
pathological.

Physiological coma is, of course, sleep. This analogy cannot be stretched too far, but there are general lessons to be learnt about coma from consideration of some of the phenomena of sleep.

Pharmacological coma is the state of surgical anaesthesia and is induced by drugs. It is possible for this type to develop into pathological coma because of maladroit administration of anaesthesia or as a result of attempts at suicide or homicide with hypnotic, sedative or narcotic drugs.

Pathological coma is that produced by systemic disease or neurological damage. There are many conditions which may on occasion result in coma, for example, diabetes mellitus, encephalitis, subarachnoid haemorrhage, cerebrovascular accidents, head injury, increased intracranial pressure and hepatic failure. This list is not complete and the differentiation between various causes of pathological coma is not discussed here.

Pathological coma and intensive therapy

The management of the comatose patient as a whole, but excluding the management of the precipitant cause, is common to all types of coma. Furthermore, much of the general management of pathological coma derives from lessons learnt from both sleep and anaesthesia.

The fact that there are so many common features of management in all the types of coma is the medico-technical reason for the development of *intensive therapy*.

Continual
Observation
Medical
Attention

is the lynch pin on which successful intensive therapy depends. Nurses and technicians, aided by various monitors and machines, provide the continual observation. The results of this process must, however, be interpreted and acted upon by specialists who are not committed elsewhere. The final stimulus which led to the development of units for intensive therapy in which to concentrate the patients, personnel and the apparatus was, of course, economic. The similarity between the management of coma and anaesthesia led inevitably and naturally to some specialists in the latter becoming closely involved with the former. A further link between the two disciplines is the common practice of induction of pharmacological coma and neuromuscular paralysis for therapeutic convenience in intensive therapy units.

Signs of coma

There are varying stages of coma which can be identified and demonstrated but in general it has become recognized that this type of categorization is unhelpful and may even be frankly misleading. Definition of the degree of pathological coma on the basis of certain physical signs is as unsatisfactory as the attempt to describe the condition of a paralysed, lightly anaesthetized patient in terms of Guedel's stages and planes of diethyl ether anaesthesia.

It is well known that the depth of physiological sleep varies through the night. The variation, or absence of variation, in the depth of general anaesthesia is under the direct control of the anaesthetist who may deepen it in order to prevent reaction to the current surgical stimulus. Surgical anaesthesia is thus not the result of the pharmacological action of drugs alone. It is the state which results when surgical stimuli are applied to a patient under the influence of anaesthetic drugs. The opposing nature of these forces should be appreciated: satisfactory anaesthesia is their resultant.

Traditionally, Guedel's classification of general anaesthesia into four stages would now be expounded; however, it is frequently irrelevant nowadays although very important historically. Modern anaesthesia in the western world does not depend upon the administration of a single agent, and certainly seldom upon open-drop diethyl ether in unpremedicated patients, which was the method on which Guedel based his classification. Premedicants, particularly the parasympatholytic drugs, the opiates and muscle relaxants all vitiate the value of the signs of the various stages of anaesthesia.

The concept that the state of general anaesthesia is demonstrated by signs of progressive depression of the central nervous system, commencing at the phylogenetically recently developed cerebral cortex and ending with medullary depression, is convenient but probably far from the truth. It used to be assumed that consciousness is a function of the cortex and that depression of the medulla is the terminal event. Consciousness is lost early in this 'journey towards death', but this is due to the effect of depression of the reticular activating system situated in the brain stem. Evidence also exists that activity of the cortex continues during apparent unconsciousness, and that the memory of this can subsequently be activated by, non-drug, hypnosis for example. It is important to understand that just as there is no single explanation of the action of all anaesthetic drugs, so there can be more than one series of signs of general anaesthesia. A few anaesthetic agents (methohexitone, enflurane, etomidate and ketamine) stimulate muscle movements which may develop into convulsions, or reveal latent epilepsy, whilst simultaneously a state of complete dissociation from the environment indistinguishable from unconsciousness results. Other agents (thiobarbiturates, ether and halothane) do not cause convulsions in the absence of hypoxia but depress consciousness without causing any excitement.

It is therefore clear that cortical *depression* is not an essential feature of pharmacological coma. The psychological importance claimed for cerebral activity during physiological sleep is well known, and it is only in pathological coma that we must assume that cerebral activity is suppressed completely.

Pathological coma is also not a steady state. The degree or depth of coma may vary considerably from hour to hour and can be considered in a generally similar manner. The patient is unresponsive to:

the spoken word,
a painful stimulus,
an increase in arterial carbon dioxide tension,
a decrease in arterial oxygen tension.

These stimuli can be progressively increased and the various responses can be used to subdivide each of the above four stages. The important principle of this type of assessment is that the response to a specific stimulus is recorded and that random records with vague qualitative terms are not employed.

Monitoring of coma

Fig. 5.1 shows a scheme for a progressive record of a patient with brain damage. The general picture of the evolution of the condition can be seen from this chart.

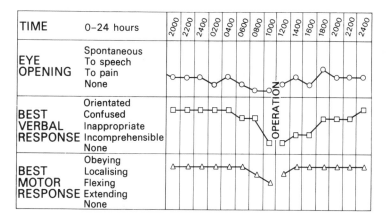

Fig. 5.1. Chart for recording assessment of consciousness. From Teasdale G. & Jennett B. (1974) *Lancet* ii, 81, with permission.

It is not surprising that the *electroencephalograph* has been used in an attempt to make assessment a little more objective. Fig. 5.2 shows one such application in the determination of prognosis in hepatic coma.

The electroencephalograph has been used similarly to separate seven levels of surgical anaesthesia and Fig. 5.3 shows a set of such traces. In contrast to the tracings in Fig. 5.2, which are of pathological coma, electroencephalographic anaesthetic level 4 is found in rapid eye movement (REM), physiological, sleep. In spite of considerable study the method has never been widely used to monitor clinical anaesthesia for surgery because of the major technical problems of the numerous electrodes, maintenance of their contact with the skin, frequency of electrical interference, to say nothing of the bulk and expense of the apparatus.

The *cerebral function monitor*, which has only two electrodes, is used to display trends in electrical output of the brain during, for instance, cardiopulmonary bypass, recovery from drug overdosage or brain damage. A drawing of a tracing from this monitor is in Fig. 5.4. A tracing represents filtered and compressed electroencephalographic outputs. Measurements of the distance of the tracing from the baseline are used for quantification of cerebral activity. Recordings of *oculomicrotremor* (fine, involuntary movement of the eyes which disappear in coma and reappear as unconsciousness lightens) are sometimes used to

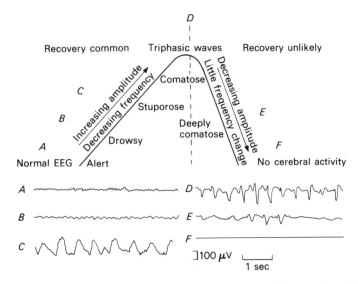

Fig. 5.2. Use of the electroencephalogram in liver failure. The records on the left of the vertical line (*A, B* and *C*) are associated commonly with recovery whilst those on the right (*E* and *F*) are uncommonly associated with recovery. From Kennedy J., Parboo S. P., MacGillaray B. & Sherlock S. (1973) *Quart. J. Med.* **167,** 54d, with permission.

assist the prognosis of coma. These movements disappear on induction of anaesthesia and reappear on recovery.

Hazards of coma

Pharmacological and pathological coma are clearly threats to life: some phenomena of sleep (snoring, postural changes and eye movements) remind us of these hazards.

The *acute* hazards are the *respiratory* ones of:
   absent protective reflexes,
   airway obstruction, and
   apnoea.

The *chronic* (long-term) hazards of coma are those of the condition and those aggravated by the therapy of the above respiratory hazards. They are related to problems with:
   secretions,
   infection,

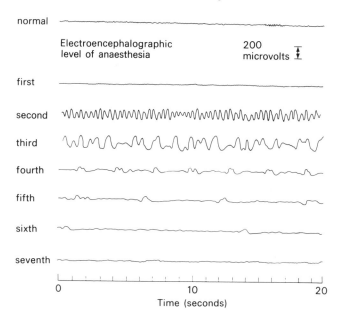

Fig. 5.3. The seven electroencephalographic levels of anaesthesia. From Courtin R. F., Bickford R. G., Faulkner A. J. (1950) *Proc. Staff Meeting Mayo Clinic* **25**, 197, with permission.

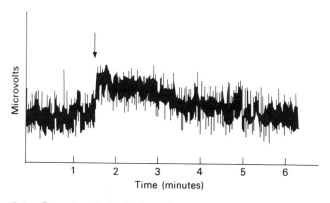

Fig. 5.4. Record at the beginning of anaesthesia from the cerebral function monitor.

nutrition,
fluid and electrolyte balance,
micturition,
pressure on the skin,
protection of the eyes,
movements of limbs,
defaecation,
the psychology and emotions of the patient and relatives.

Sleep, although physiological, is also associated in some pathological circumstances with hazards from apnoea and airway obstruction. Recent interest and research has confirmed that the parallels between the three types of coma are not so far fetched as some thought.

Absent protective reflexes

Total absence of protective reflexes is an extreme condition and occurs only in deep coma. The laryngeal reflex which results in a cough is normally initiated by inhalation of foreign material or mucus. This cough may be depressed by drugs or disease, but coughing still occurs when the carina at the bifurcation of the trachea is stimulated. Ciliary activity is depressed by morphine and by general anaesthetic drugs, with the result that when foreign material reaches the bronchi it is less likely to be wafted back towards the larynx.

Some inhaled general anaesthetics (diethyl ether, isoflurane) are irritant to the larynx and bronchi and stimulate reflex activity. They also cause increased secretions from the mucus-secreting glands of these areas. Sudden increases in inspired concentrations can cause the larynx partially to close - laryngeal stridor - during inspiration. Laryngeal spasm is an extreme form of this condition which can persist until the hypoxaemia which results causes it to relax or until anaesthesia is much more profound.

Depression of the respiratory reflexes is progressive. Loss of airway protective reflexes occurs early. Loss of the ability to overcome the effects of an inadequate airway (airway obstruction) occurs next. Apnoea, which is the manifestation of the loss of the rhythmic breathing reflex, is the final stage.

Management has to be combined with the management of established airway obstruction, or its prophylaxis, and apnoea (see later). There are a few special situations in which more or less specific therapy can be employed but these drugs are not appropriate in all cases of coma.

Narcotic antagonists should be administered to patients who are unconscious from narcotic overdosage. If there is any doubt about the nature of the drug causing depression, naloxone, which is free from agonist activity, is the drug of choice. Its action is, however, brief and depression of ventilation recurs. The other narcotic antagonists, nalorphine and levallorphan, themselves cause depression if no narcotic is already present and they are longer acting.

Doxapram is a *respiratory stimulant* which acts directly on the carotid bodies to stimulate ventilation. It is effective in the presence of narcotics but, unlike the narcotic antagonists, has no action upon the analgesic effect. It is therefore a useful drug in the postoperative period.

Physostigmine is an *analeptic* drug and acts centrally as a cholinesterase inhibitor. In contrast to other similar inhibitors it is a tertiary amine and can therefore cross the blood-brain barrier. The action of some long-acting sedatives, particularly the diazepines, can be terminated promptly with this drug. Aminophylline is another non specific respiratory stimulant/agonist to diazepines which may be used, but there is a specific antagonist to these drugs under development.

There is evidence that laryngeal reflexes are impaired for some hours after general anaesthesia even though recovery appears to be complete. Oral intake of fluids should start with a few sips of water. Large volumes straightaway are likely to cause the patient to vomit, but provided intake is gradually increased there is no need to withhold fluids for a long time.

Airway obstruction

This commonly occurs in all types of coma. It can be:

    partial, or

    complete.

Partial airway obstruction is colloquially referred to as snoring. This is due on most occasions to the tongue which falls backwards on to the posterior pharyngeal wall so that the soft palate is caused to vibrate more than usual as a result of the rapid flow of gas through the narrowed channel. The tongue is mostly muscle and is relaxed during unconsciousness or when skeletal muscle relaxants have been used. Involuntary snoring during lectures often awakens the student who immediately corrects the inadequate airway. Conscious subjects do not usually snore.

Other causes of partial airway obstruction are:

    oral secretions,

    food,

vomit,
misplaced dentures,
blood, and
tumours.

Fig. 5.5 shows how the tongue causes partial airway obstruction.

The *signs* of partial airway obstruction are often audible and there is increased respiratory effort in the attempt to overcome the obstruction, but reduced volumes of air are exchanged in relation to this effort. The diaphragm moves downwards more vigorously than usual during inspiration so that the abdominal wall is forced outwards. (This tends to follow after the movement of the chest and is sometimes erroneously referred to as paradoxical respiration. It is not.) The intercostal muscles contribute to the increased effort and the accessory muscles of respiration (sternomastoid, platysma, trapezius) may be active. The alae nasi dilate during inspiration.

These vigorous respiratory movements are responsible for one of the most serious hazards of the condition. When the diaphragm moves downwards the cardiac 'sphincter' becomes less efficient in the prevention of retrograde emptying of the stomach. Furthermore, because of

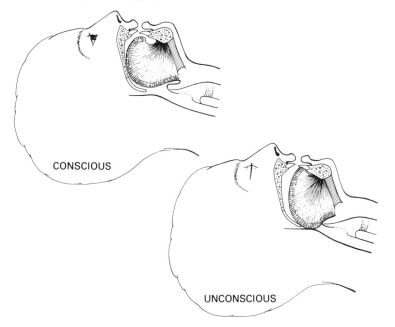

CONSCIOUS

UNCONSCIOUS

Fig. 5.5. The position of the tongue and jaw in a conscious and unconsious supine subject.

the movement downards of the diaphragm, the intragastric pressure is raised. Gastric contents may thus be *regurgitated* into the pharynx. If the laryngeal reflexes were also impaired it is likely that the next violent inspiration may cause some of this material to be sucked into the major airways. Alternatively, if regurgitation were to happen fortuitously just before correction of the upper airway, aspiration might again occur. Aspiration can also occur in the elderly even when the laryngeal reflex is not depressed by drugs or disease. Asphyxiation follows or, if the material is fluid, widespread pulmonary damage.

Another hazard of the vigorous respiratory efforts is that the increased subatmospheric pressure in the intrapleural space may be sufficient to overcome the osmotic pressure in the alveolar capillaries, and cause fluid to be drawn into the alveolar spaces with the result that *pulmonary oedema* develops.

Hypercapnia is a fairly late development because although increased alveolar ventilation is the first response to accumulation of carbon dioxide this only later decreases so that carbon dioxide is retained. The signs of this condition are described in Chapter 7.

Hypoxia, particularly when the patient is breathing air, is common. Mucous membranes and the skin become cyanosed or blue, pulse rate and arterial blood pressure increase and the respiratory efforts become more vigorous. The conscious patient is usually acutely anxious and this only serves to aggravate the effects of the condition.

Hypoxia causes restlessness. Sedatives, hypnotics or analgesics should NEVER be prescribed. The patient must receive controlled oxygen therapy.

The *clinical signs of an adequate normal airway* are:
    rhythmic, unlaboured, quiet respiration,
    synchronous movement of the chest and abdomen,
    palpable expiration (with the palm of the observer's hand),
    pink colour of mucous membranes,
    absence of signs of airway obstruction.

Management of airway obstruction is a most important skill for an undergraduate to acquire

The airway must be cleared of foreign matter and the tongue manipulated away from the posterior pharyngeal wall. This may be achieved in three ways which are not mutually exclusive:
    elevate the lower jaw,
    insert a pharyngeal airway,
    place the patient in the coma position.

The tongue is moved forwards by all three of these manoeuvres. Fig. 5.6 shows the effect of elevation of the lower jaw upon the airway. Sometimes this is achieved by holding the mandible at the symphysis mentis but on other occasions both angles of the mandible must be firmly pushed forwards. Fig. 5.7 shows how to insert a pharyngeal airway correctly.

The *coma position* is recognized throughout the world as a safe one for unconscious patients.

In Fig. 5.8 the patient is lying left side down with the right leg over the left in order to prevent further pronation on to the face. The back can either be supported with a pillow or the left arm can be pulled underneath the chest so that it prevents the movement of supination. The left-hand side tends to be recommended by anaesthetists since conventional laryngoscopes are designed to push the tongue to the left and gravity helps rather than hinders if the patient's head is already on the left. The right-hand side may however have advantages because it is regularly demonstrated in departments of radiology that stomach emptying occurs more rapidly when patients lie on the right rather than on the left side.

If vomiting occurs in an unconscious subject, drainage from the mouth is improved by this posture and the risk of a threat to the laryngeal inlet with its impaired sensitivity is lessened.

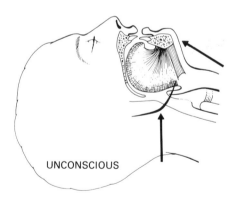

Fig. 5.6. The effect of raising the jaw on the position of the tongue of a supine, unconscious subject. The arrows indicate the two sites at which the manoeuvre of elevation can be achieved.

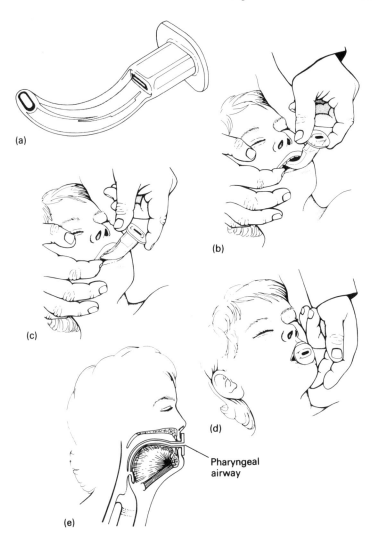

(a)

(b)

(c)

(d)

(e)

Pharyngeal
airway

Fig. 5.7a An oropharyngeal airway.
Fig. 5.7b—d Insertion of this airway into a patient's mouth. Note that it is put in upside down until the tip is well over the tongue and it is then rotated (5.7c) and pushed over the back of the tongue. Notice that throughout this manoeuvre the anaesthetist is maintaining the airway with one hand.
Fig. 5.7e The pharyngeal airway supporting the tongue.

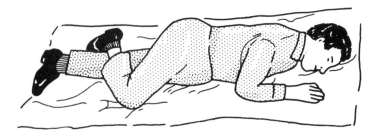

Fig. 5.8. The coma position. The left (under) arm is preventing the subject rolling backwards and the right knee and right arm are preventing forward rotation.

All postoperative patients who are unconscious should be placed in the coma position. If bleeding in the mouth following dental extraction or upper airway surgery is a risk, the head can be placed lower than the chest.

Complete airway obstruction. Asphyxiation and death occurs very rapidly once partial airway obstruction becomes complete. Sudden death by drowning, aspiration of food (which sometimes follows vomiting or occurs during mastication), haemorrhage into the respiratory tract and electrocution are all possible independent causes.

The *signs* of complete airway obstruction are those of partial obstruction except that no air can be felt or heard to pass the upper airway, and the efforts of ventilation become increasingly violent. The patient rapidly becomes intensely cyanosed and sweats profusely. Anxiety is promptly replaced by acute panic because the patient is fully aware of the situation when the condition has been progressive. Consciousness is soon lost.

Emergency management of acute airway obstruction should be within the capability of all citizens. Drainage of fluid material can be encouraged by putting the victim head down and sometimes solid substances can be dislodged from their position by a sharp blow on the back. When a child inhales a solid lump of food this action is frequently effective. Smaller objects (tooth, pea or peanut) often cause serious problems when they reach their eventual resting place in a major (usually the right) bronchus.

The *Heimlich manoeuvre* (Fig. 5.9) is one method of dislodgement of inhaled solids which is effective. The rescuer strikes the victim sharply

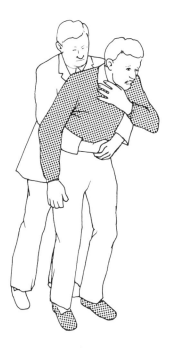

Fig. 5.9. The Heimlich manoeuvre.

in the abdomen just below the ribs in an upward and backwards direction. The sudden egress of air acts as a forceful artificial cough.

Relief of complete airway obstruction in hospital is frequently unsuccessful. The above measures are carried out first but if they fail intubation of the trachea and tracheal suction should be attempted. Bronchoscopy is performed only for lower airway obstruction and is rarely required as a life-saving manoeuvre.

When the obstruction is in the mouth, pharynx or larynx, intubation may be difficult or impossible. Urgent tracheotomy (*cut* in the trachea) can be performed. Alternatively, a wide-bore (2-3 mm) needle can be thrust into the airway just above or just below the cricoid cartilage. Sufficient oxygen can be caused to flow through this to enable adequate oxygenation to occur. The Minitrach (Fig. 5.10) is a device to facilitate this manoeuvre. Definitive *tracheostomy* (surgically fashioned opening, *-ostomy*) can be performed later.

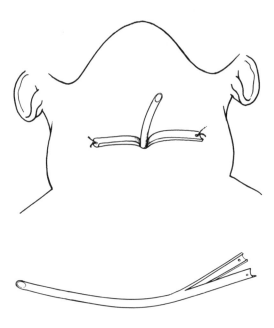

Fig. 5.10.   The Minitrach.

Apnoea

This is the preterminal condition of coma. It is caused by acute or acute on chronic neurological defect following brain damage or by overdosage of drugs.

Carbon dioxide accumulates so that the arterial tension rises by about 0.4–0.6 kPa (3–5 mm Hg) per minute. Hypoxia develops rapidly and within 2 minutes of apnoea the arterial oxygen tension is likely to have declined to 5.3 kPa (40 mmHg) when apnoea follow air-breathing.

The *signs* are that no respiratory effort is made and expiration cannot be felt with the observer's hand. It may very occasionally be difficult to observe shallow ventilation.

Management. Controlled ventilation must be established as soon as possible (see Chapter 8).

Monitoring in anaesthesia
(pharmacological coma)

Anaesthetists induce coma, with all its attendant risks, in patients so that their surgical operations are painless. Pharmacological coma is entirely different in this respect from all others: it is intentional, not accidental and it is drug-induced, not physiological.

Since the risk-ridden state of anaesthesia has been purposely caused it should be carefully and regularly assessed. Deterioration in the patient's condition must be detected early so that remedial action can be instituted. This process is called monitoring (Latin *moneo*, I warn). Some observations are made continuously and others are intermittent. Repeated regular measurements can inform the anaesthetist and others of the imminence of change more effectively than qualitative opinions unsupported by measurements.

Monitoring of the anaesthetic state is, as already mentioned, seldom achieved during routine operations by electrophysiological measurements. There is no machine which enables the patients to say to the anaesthetist, 'I am adequately anaesthetized for this operation'.

The following clinical signs are sought by the anaesthetist and used as indicators of light anaesthesia:

lacrimation,
reflex movement,
pupillary dilatation,
hypertension,
tachycardia, and
sweating.

These signs are by no means pathognomic since similar signs may occur in many different circumstances such as:

hypercapnia,
following direct stimulation of nerves,
when ambient temperature is increased,
over transfusion,
hypoxia, or
increased circulating endogenous catecholamines.

(Lacrimation is not a constant sign of light anaesthesia and is partly inhibited by atropine, but lacrimal secretion is not the response in any of the other conditions.)

It is important to remember that the last special sense to be depressed is hearing: conversation and movement should therefore be quiet. It is likely that further sensory deprivation can be provided by the use of ear plugs.

Physiological monitoring

Many of the early developments of physiological monitoring in intensive therapy units were derived directly from the experience of monitoring in the operating room.

Respiratory monitoring

This includes observation and/or measurement of:

the concentration of the inspired gases,
ventilatory volumes,
and the effect of ventilation.

The concentration of the inspired gases in a one-way system (see Chapter 3) may be calculated from the flow meter readings.

Many anaesthetic systems allow some rebreathing of expired gas and are not unidirectional. The only method under these circumstances is actually to measure the concentration of gases. The usual gas to be measured is oxygen and there are several different types of analyser designed to achieve this. Interpretation of arterial blood gas analysis is impossible unless the inspired oxygen concentration is known accurately (see Chapter 7).

Continuous, breath-by-breath, recordings of changes of gas concentrations can be made with rapid response infrared analysers (capnographs for carbon dioxide) or with mass spectrometers for physiological (oxygen and carbon dioxide) and anaesthetic gases.

This type of measurement is extremely useful because, not only is information obtained about the inspired concentrations of carbon dioxide for example, but also the efficiency of the ventilation in the elimination of carbon dioxide can be assessed. Fig. 5.11 shows a capnograph tracing of an anaesthetized, paralysed and ventilated patient. It can be seen that the inspired carbon dioxide concentration is 2% and that the maximum concentration at the end of expiration is just over 5%. This end-expiratory carbon dioxide concentration is very close to the alveolar concentration which, in turn, is close to the arterial level. Notice that despite the fact that carbon dioxide is inhaled the arterial carbon dioxide is not raised. This efficient elimination of carbon dioxide indicates that alveolar ventilation is satisfactory.

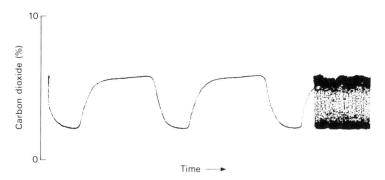

Fig. 5.11. The concentration of carbon dioxide at the lips of a patient receiving controlled ventilation with some rebreathing. See text.

Fig. 5.12 is a similar tracing: notice that the slope of the tracing continues to rise and when the next inspiration is imposed by the automatic ventilator the highest concentration *might* not yet have been reached. This is the phenomenon of maldistribution. No confident deduction is possible about the alveolar concentration of carbon dioxide from this record because it is clear that carbon dioxide elimination has not yet ceased, and were expiration to continue the concentration might rise further.

Mass spectrometry can be used in a similar manner to provide breath-by-breath analysis of all the other respired gases. These instruments are at present mainly used in research departments, but have great potential in intensive therapy units. Other analysers are sometimes used for gases and vapours other than carbon dioxide and oxygen but they have no application outside the operating room.

Ventilatory volumes. Observation of the movements of the reservoir bag coupled with those of the patient's chest is an important *qualitative* monitor (see Chapter 3) of spontaneous ventilation. If a disparity exists, that is very little movement of the reservoir bag but larger movements of the chest, airway obstruction or a large leak in the system may be suspected.

Stethoscopy, oesophageal or chest wall, is another simple monitor.

The above approaches are the traditional ones used in countless operating rooms. They do not permit easy communication from one person to another and cannot always be used effectively. Quantitative measurements of total ventilation are gradually taking their place.

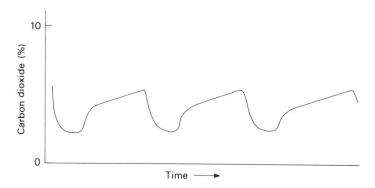

Fig. 5.12. The concentration of carbon dioxide at the lips from a patient showing maldistribution. See text.

There are a number of different ways to *measure* the volume of ventilation. When a non-return anaesthetic system is in use the total fresh gas flow in litres/min equals the minute ventilation of the patient, provided that there is no leak from the system and that the reservoir bag is neither exhausted of gas nor progressively distended.

Direct measurements are provided by spirometers of several different designs and can be used during both spontaneous and controlled ventilation. Many of these are unidirectional. It is important, therefore, to check that the spirometer has been correctly positioned before assuming malfunction. It is usual to measure expired ventilation on the assumption that the volume expired *must* have been inspired. The converse is not necessarily true.

These measurements are of total ventilation. Alveolar ventilation may be as little as half the total ventilation during controlled ventilation and anaesthesia owing to increases in physiological dead space. Conscious young adults waste about 30% of total ventilation but under anaesthesia, muscular paralysis and controlled ventilation this may increase by 10%. Older people, both because of their age and because of intercurrent chronic disease may waste as much as 60% of the total ventilation under the same conditions. Thus spirometry of total ventilation can provide only an approximate idea about the adequacy of alveolar ventilation.

The *results* or *effects of ventilation* are on the oxygen and carbon dioxide levels in arterial blood. These are expressed as arterial tensions, that is to say, the partial pressure of gas with which the arterial blood has reached equilibrium. Gas flows as a result of a pressure difference:

thus, since arterial oxygen tension is greater than tissue oxygen tension, oxygen moves towards tissue. (Tension is used in the liquid phase (blood) and partial pressure in the gaseous phase (alveolar). The French word *tension* means pressure: P is the international symbol for tension or partial pressure of gas.)

The carbon dioxide tension in arterial blood ($PaCO_2$) is inversely related to the alveolar ventilation (V_A) provided that carbon dioxide production is constant. (Strictly this relationship relates alveolar carbon dioxide and alveolar ventilation but arterial and alveolar tensions can be considered as the same for this particular purpose.)

Thus,

$$PaCO_2 = k \times \frac{1}{V_A}$$

(where k includes carbon dioxide output and those constants required to convert carbon dioxide concentration to partial pressure).

This is approximately linear over most of the clinical range of alveolar ventilation and carbon dioxide tension so that halving one value doubles the other. It does not apply at very high arterial carbon dioxide tensions when alveolar ventilation is depressed by the anaesthetic action of carbon dioxide. Carbon dioxide output is, of course, lower during anaesthesia and during hypothermia than it is in the conscious state.

The arterial carbon dioxide tension is lowered by hyperventilation: the lungs of many patients are so ventilated and values of 3.3–4.0 kPa (25–30 mmHg) are not unusual. It should be remembered that the carbon dioxide tension is an important determinant of:

    cerebral blood flow,
    oxyhaemoglobin dissociation,
    hydrogen ion activity, and
    cardiac output.

The relationship with *cerebral blood flow* is linear and if the arterial carbon dioxide tension is doubled so is the cerebral blood flow. Hyperventilation is deliberately employed in neurosurgery, but a reduction of 25–30% in cerebral blood flow might be critical in a patient with cerebral atherosclerosis during other surgery.

The *association of haemoglobin with oxygen* is reduced by an increase in arterial carbon dioxide but dissociation is increased. Uptake of oxygen in the lungs is reduced but delivery of oxygen at the tissues is increased. Another way of expressing the same fact is to say that the oxyhaemoglobin dissociation is moved to the right and the P_{50} is increased. (The P_{50} is defined as that tension of oxygen when the haemoglobin is 50% saturated with oxygen.)

The importance of carbon dioxide in determining the *hydrogen ion activity* (pH) of the blood is well known. Acute changes in arterial carbon dioxide tension are unlikely to exceed the buffering capacity of the blood and pH changes are thus not common. However, changes in pH affect drug activity and it is important that they are avoided.

Cardiac output declines by 1% for each 0.133 kPa (1 mmHg) reduction in arterial carbon dioxide tension. If a normal patient were to be maximally hyperventilated during anaesthesia to an arterial carbon dioxide tension of 3.3 kPa (25 mmHg), the cardiac output (say 3.5 litres/min under anaesthesia) decreases by a further 15%, which is 525 ml/min.

Each of the above four changes are important to an anaesthetized patient and may be critical in sick patients. The constant attention by anaesthetists to ventilation is thus justified.

The arterial carbon dioxide tension is raised during hypoventilation. Arterial hypertension and serious dysrhythmias may follow (see pages 91–3 and Chapter 7).

Oxygenation is also affected by anaesthesia and an account of the physiology involved is given later in Chapter 7. Hypoxia is not inevitable and is avoided by a number of manoeuvres described there.

Arterial cannulation cannot be performed ethically in all patients receiving general anaesthesia, but the information from continuous blood pressure recordings and blood gas analysis of occasionally repeated samples is invaluable during major surgery. It is from information derived from such use that general lessons can be learnt and the practice of anaesthesia made more safe for all patients.

Cardiovascular monitoring

Measurement of systolic blood pressure by indirect methods and counting the pulse rate are the commonest means used by anaesthetists to monitor the cardiovascular system but there are limitations to these measurements which should be understood.

When the surgical procedure is such that serious haemorrhage frequently occurs, intermittent or better still continuous, direct recordings of arterial and central venous pressures should be made. An example of such a recording is given in Fig. 5.13. Notice the effect of controlled ventilation upon both the central venous and the arterial blood press-

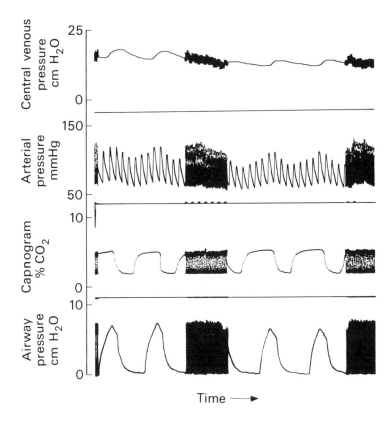

Fig. 5.13. Simultaneous tracing recorded during a general anaesthetic including controlled ventilation. See text.

ures. This amounts to variations of 20 mmHg in systolic arterial and 2.5 cmH$_2$O in central venous blood pressures.

Knowledge about the *pressure* of blood in the supply vessels does not convey information to the observer about the *flow* of blood through the tissue which is supplied. It is nevertheless this flow which determines the delivery of oxygen. Vasoconstriction may result in a high driving pressure but poor perfusion: vasodilatation may, on occasion, be followed by improved perfusion although the driving pressure may be relatively low.

There are several indirect methods of judging the quality of *organ perfusion*. These are:

capillary refill,
colour,
temperature,
biological electrical potentials,
organ function.

Capillary refill, i.e. the refilling with blood of capillaries in the skin or mucous membranes after the removal of pressure applied to blanch the tissue, is supposed to indicate adequacy of perfusion. It is clear that, whilst organ perfusion may be satisfactory, that through the skin may not be; the converse may also happen.

The *colour* of the blood which refills capillaries is affected by ambient temperature and thus many anaesthetists tend to observe capillary refill on the buccal (inside) surface of the lips. Others attempt to abolish the effects of temperature by rubbing the surface of the skin or by the observation of capillary refill in nail-beds.

The *temperature* of a peripheral surface is usually lower than that of the core of the body. A poorly perfused tissue is cold and vice versa. Fig. 5.14 demonstrates the difference betwen core temperature and the peripheral (finger) temperature in a patient with a perforated peptic ulcer. Fluid replacement caused a gradual decline in this difference and

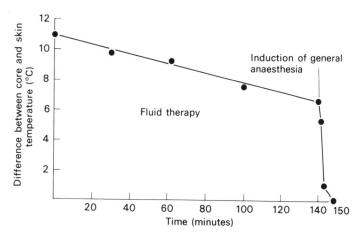

Fig. 5.14. Gradual reduction of the difference between core temperature and skin temperature as fluid therapy progresses: note the sudden abolition of this difference on induction of general anaesthesia.

when vasodilatation took place at the induction of anaesthesia the difference abruptly disappeared.

Biological potentials emanating from some muscle tissue and from the brain are amplified and displayed as electromyographs, electrocardiographs and electroncephalographs. These tracings do not indicate that the perfusion of the organs in which the potentials are created is optimal, but they do indicate that the organs are perfused. It is certainly true to say that when there is no perfusion the tracings disappear, although there may be a delay of a few seconds before this occurs.

Organ function must continue if perfusion continues. If that specific function can be monitored it is the best noninvasive indicator available of adequate perfusion. *Urine production* cannot take place unless blood flows through the kidney. The quality of the urine secreted need not be perfect but the fact that it is secreted must imply that blood is traversing the kidney. The kidneys are the only splanchnic organs whose function can be assessed continually during anaesthesia. It is assumed that, if renal blood flow is adequate, then perfusion of other organs is also adequate.

The above arguments might suggest that peripheral perfusion is the sole factor in assessing normality of cardiovascular function. It is not; adequacy of the cardiac pump is another important variable.

Cardiac output is also assessed indirectly by observation of several different variables:

> capillary refill time,
> temperature,
> systolic arterial pressure,
> central venous pressure,
> pulse rate.

The *time* which elapses from release of pressure and the return of perfusion must reflect the value of the cardiac output. A brief interval suggests normal or increased cardiac output and adequate peripheral vascular tone. Sluggish return indicates decreased cardiac output.

A cool peripheral *temperature* indicates vasoconstriction and, under some circumstances, indicates a low cardiac output. For example in the absence of peripheral vascular disease and in the presence of an appropriate recent history, immediately following cardiopulmonary bypass for instance, a large difference between the central core temperature and the periphery is commonly interpreted as an indicator of a low cardiac output. The vasoconstriction gradually relaxes over a few hours after bypass and this, in conjunction with other changes, indicates an increase in cardiac output.

The limitations of *arterial blood pressure* have already been mentioned: an isolated, normal or near normal value does not indicate an adequate cardiac output. The value of the *central venous pressure* (see below) is not by itself very informative about cardiac output and, in any case, only refers to the right side of the heart (see Chapter 7).

The *pulse rate*, and the baroreceptor reflexes which influence it, are affected by anaesthesia. However, so long as complete beta-adrenergic blockade has not been instituted, an increase in pulse rate still takes place when cardiac output decreases.

Assessment of cardiac output is a matter of summation of all the available information. Each of the variables used in the assessment of peripheral perfusion have their own importance but when they are used to assess cardiac output they must all be considered simultaneously.

Cardiac output may, on occasion, be measured directly. The invasive methods involve cannulation of both an artery and of a central vein or cannulation of the pulmonary artery (see page 115). Each of these cannulations may be responsible for morbidity and they are not therefore employed without careful consideration. A recent, indirect, non-invasive method for the observation of trends in cardiac output is to record the changes in electrical impedance across the chest.

Central venous pressure

This is the pressure in the great veins or right atrium and it represents the filling pressure of the right heart. It is best measured by means of a catheter passed via a peripheral vein. Fig. 5.15 shows the arrangement commonly employed. The units of pressure are usually cmH_2O because these are the units actually employed in the technique of measurement (but, more rationally, in departments of cardiology mmHg are used). Cannulae in large veins (external jugular) are occasionally used to monitor changes in central venous pressure provided that venous valves do not interfere with the pressure recorded. Confirmation that the end of the catheter is within the chest should be sought by radiograph. Catheters can pass into the most unlikely sites when they are inserted blindly. The presence of swings in pressure associated with respiration is confirmatory but not conclusive evidence that a satisfactory position has been obtained. Central venous and systolic arterial pressure readings are affected by intrathoracic pressure and may therefore appear

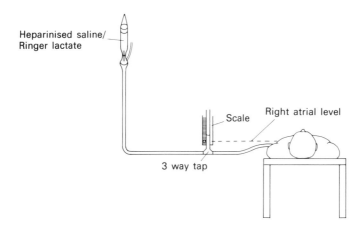

Heparinised saline/
Ringer lactate

Scale

Right atrial level

3 way tap

Fig. 5.15. The arrangement of the flushing solution and manometer for the determination of central venous pressure.

to be raised during intermittent positive pressure ventilation (see Fig. 5.13).

Determination of the central venous pressure is not an end in itself. Rarely, if ever, are isolated readings of value. Trends, in association with trends in systolic arterial blood pressure and pulse rate, are useful when dynamic changes are taking place. Fig. 5.16 indicates idealized examples of the four possible combinations of trends in central venous and systolic arterial pressure which are seen.

Electrocardiograph

This important monitor should always be employed. Electrodes can be placed quickly and remotely from the site of surgery and reliable, convenient, display apparatus is now widely available. The differential diagnosis of cardiac arrest depends on the use of this monitor (see Chapter 8); the clinical diagnosis can be made without it. Disturbances of cardiac rhythm can, however, only be recognized confidently with its aid. Many dysrhythmias which occur under anaesthesia have significant haemodynamic effects.

Atrial nodal rhythm is one common dysrhythmia: it is seldom important but sometimes it causes systolic hypotension. Fig. 5.17 shows the effect of intravenous atropine on this: both the dysrhythmia and the

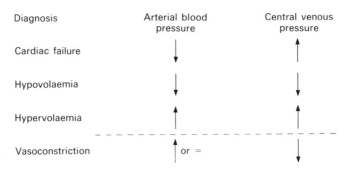

Fig. 5.16. Directions of the combined trends of central venous and arterial blood pressures with their appropriate diagnostic interpretations. The changes of vasoconstriction are seldom seen in the conscious patient but are very occasionally witnessed under anaesthesia.

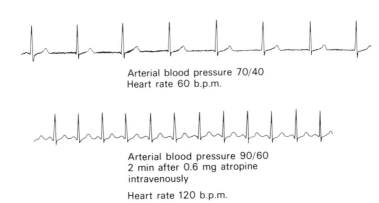

Fig. 5.17. Atrial nodal rhythm with haemodynamic consequences treated with atropine.

hypotension were immediately reversed. Occasional ventricular ectopic beats are also common and relatively unimportant. However, when these become frequent, hypotension and myocardial hypoxia are the result and ventricular fibrillation may follow. A high inspired concentration of halothane is one common cause of both these dysrhythmias, which are initially benign, and early warning following observation of an electrocardiograph prevents the need for emergency treatment.

Another example of the importance of the level of arterial carbon dioxide tension and dysrhythmias is given in Fig. 5.18. This is an

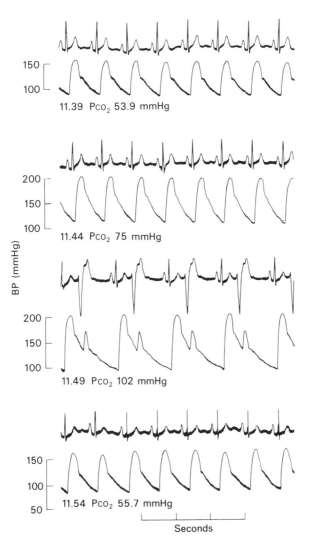

Fig. 5.18. Hypercapnia associated with hypertension and a dysrhythmia. From Payne J. P. (1962) *Acta Scand. Anaesth.* **6,** 129, with permission.

historic record because the technique of anaesthesia during which it was obtained is now regarded by most anaesthetists as unsafe, but the illustration which it provides is valuable.

Finally, the shape of the electrocardiographic trace, particularly the ST segment, may indicate myocardial ischaemia and indicate to the anaesthetist the need for a change in management.

Blood volume monitoring

Changes in blood volume, particularly hypovolaemia, are detected by observation of a number of physiological variables (arterial and venous pressures, pulse rate, peripheral vascular tone: see earlier but the volumes of blood actually in, or physically lost from, the circulation are seldom measured accurately during an operation. Wet swabs may be weighed and the increase in weight over the dry weight is assumed to be related to the blood loss. Large volumes of blood may be collected in suckers but the insiduous losses of small volumes are often missed.

The anaesthetic record

An example is shown in Figure 5.19. Regular recordings are made in order that changes and trends are readily detected by the anaesthetist and that, in the event of a subsequent misadventure or complication, there is a clear account of all events and of all drugs used during the operation to which reference may easily be made. The record may usefully be continued in the recovery room.

Students should familiarize themselves with anaesthetic records since many early postoperative events can be readily interpreted from the information which is recorded there, much to the benefit of the patient.

Neuromuscular monitoring

Development of paralysing agents used by anaesthetists during the last 40 years accelerated in the late 1970's, and several drugs emerged whose actions were significantly different from those of their forbears. The emphasis of research was directed towards rapidity of onset and offset. Success in this effort resulted in an even greater requirement than before for anaesthetists to be able to measure both the degree and the duration of neuromuscular paralysis.

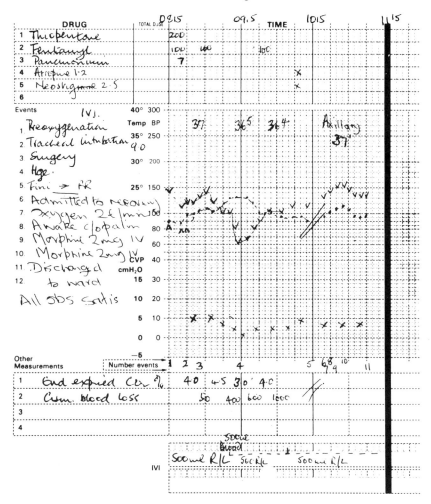

Fig. 5.19. The anaesthetic record.

The early neuromuscular blocking agents had slow onset times and very gradual offset times. Tubocurarine, and subsequently pancuronium, which despite some disadvantages were favourite drugs, required to be reversed at the end of the operation and the use of both was occasionally associated with *recurarization* some time after apparently satisfactory recovery of neuromuscular function. One of the newer drugs, vecuronium, has, not only a briefer action than these, but also its offset time, with or without reversal with anticholinesterase drugs, is less. Atracurium, destroyed *in vivo* by Hofmann elimination (non-enzymatic degradation in the blood) has similar actions. The action of both drugs during anaesthesia may cease very suddenly. The anaesthetist needs to be forewarned of this event and monitoring of neuromuscular function is essential for quality anaesthesia.

There are several approaches to this problem: all depend upon stimulation of a motor nerve and the detection of contraction of muscles either by eye, palpation or by a force transducer. Electromyography is also used. Possibly the most reliable of these is the *train-of-four* response which is a record of the response to four, timed stimuli and a comparison is made of the fourth with the first response.

The place of monitoring instruments

The detailed way in which this subject has been treated indicates its importance to the medical student. Careful observation, where necessary aided by appropriate instruments, is essential for the proper management of all patients who are unconscious irrespective of how they reached that state. Each of the methods described in this chapter is applied in the operating room and many have since found their place in the intensive care and resuscitation wards, coronary care and special baby care units. Anaesthetists are often found in these locations too.

Instruments can never replace human observations completely but they do help, particularly in the long term management of very ill patients. Equipment is now becoming more and more reliable and certainly does not become fatigued or distracted from its task by extraneous factors. It is vital however for those responsible for patient care *always to remember to look first at the patient* to check that all is well and then, in the event of an alarm signal from an instrument, to seek the fault there.

6. Pharmacology in anaesthetics: local and regional analgesia

The deposition of a local analgesic drug close to a mixed nerve, a nerve root, amongst a plexus of nerves or ganglia, or in the cerebrospinal fluid, constitutes the practice of local analgesia. It is a meeting point between many different specialists and, is sometimes quite wrongly, a focus of disagreement. *Local analgesia can be practised by any specialist provided that the dangers of both method and drugs are fully understood, and that the management of complications, should they arise, are within his practical competence.* Nevertheless, the general use of these methods is a specific part of the practice of an anaesthetist.

Mode of action

All the drugs known as local analgesic drugs have a common structure with lipophilic and hydrophilic elements which are separated and linked by an amide or an ester. The axon membrane has a similar structure: the outer layers are hydrophilic, the inner layers lipophilic. It is suggested that local analgesics are orientated similarly around their site of action. Both elements of the structure share in that anaesthetic action.

Local analgesics alter the function of the axon membrane; they also affect any excitable tissue including striated and unstriated muscle. The resting potential is unaffected but depolarization is prevented by concentrations of drug which produce a block. When that concentration is not quite great enough to do this, the threshold for excitation is increased, the impulse propagation is slowed and the rise of action potential is decreased.

Most local analgesics are weak bases. They are formulated, for pharmaceutical reasons of stability and solubility, as salts. Both the cationic form of the local analgesic salt and the un-ionized base are effective. Thus the effects of changes in hydrogen ion activity are not straightforward. Increase in the un-ionized fraction by tissue acidosis increases penetrance but may decrease duration of action. The phenomena that repeated doses of local analgesic result in tachyphylaxis, and that adrenaline decreases tissue perfusion and therefore the removal of drug, are both partly explained by the fact that an increase in hydrogen ion activity occurs as a result of both these processes.

97

Table 6.1   Relationship between size and function of nerve fibres

		Fibre size	Conduction	Onset of block
A	Myelinated. Somatic	Large	Rapid	
α	motor, proprioception,			6th
β	touch			5th
γ	muscle spindle			4th
d	pain, temperature			3rd
B	Myelinated. Autonomic	$\downarrow$	$\downarrow$	1st
C	Non-myelinated. Pain, temperature	Small	Slow	2nd

Table 6.1 shows a simplified classification of nerve fibres. The finer fibres are blocked first; recovery occurs in the reverse order.

Comparison of the relative efficacy of local analgesics is possible by means of minimum concentration (CM) which is that necessary to block conduction in a fibre of stated diameter. Thick fibres have a larger CM than fine fibres. Thus motor fibres are blocked later than pain fibres and by higher concentrations of analgesic.

Sensory block of mixed nerves occurs when the concentration of local analgesic around the nerve is lower than that required to cause motor block. Sensory fibres in the mantle of a limb nerve emanate from the proximal distribution of that nerve and those in the core of the nerve from the periphery. Therefore analgesic effects tend to be observed first in the proximal areas.

It is customary to describe the effect of local analgesics in terms of:
onset time,
intensity,
duration.
These variables are in turn related to:
mass movement of drug,
diffusion,
blood flow.

Types of local analgesia

These are:
Surface (eye, nose, pharynx, larynx, urethra)
Infiltration

Nerve
Ganglion
Plexus
Epidural (cervical, thoracic, lumbar, sacral (caudal) routes)
Spinal
Intravenous

Table 6.2   Potential (practical) sites for regional analgesia

Nerve	Digital	Dorsal nerves of penis
	Median	Ilio-inguinal
	Ulnar	Genitofemoral
	Sciatic	Supraorbital
	Femoral	Inferior dental
	Obturator	
Ganglia		
	Trigeminal	
	Gasserian	
	Stellate	
	Lumbar sympathetic	
Plexus		
	Cervical	
	Brachial	
	Coeliac	

Table 6.2 lists some of the nerves, ganglia and plexuses which are sometimes blocked. These are not all frequently performed to produce surgical anaesthesia but they are employed in the management of pain. The table indicates the potential of regional analgesia for surgical purposes where other considerations preclude general anaesthesia, but many are combined with general anaesthesia for the management of postoperative pain.

Three techniques of local analgesia are described which any doctor might find useful.

Infiltration analgesia

This is not often relevant to the practice of anaesthetists and is usually performed by the operator. The commonest causes of failure are:

inappropriate drug,
inadequate dosage,
inadequate patience.

A large volume of dilute local analgesic solution can sometimes separate tissue planes and reduce bleeding. The solution should be systematically deposited first in the superficial layers and then more deeply, and time must be allowed for the drug to work. An incision should not be made until at least one minute after injection of the drug, otherwise failure is inevitable. Sometimes it is better to use a specific nerve block (e.g. supraorbital for scalp lacerations) than to use an otherwise imprecise method. One puncture of the skin and the careful use of a long fine needle avoids repeated injections. It is wise for any practitioner to be aware of the maximum safe dose of local anaesthetic, to know how to manage both anaphylaxis and systemic effects and to consult with an anaesthetist beforehand (see pages 102–4).

Surface analgesia

This method can readily be used on mucous membranes of:
  nose,
  gums,
  eye,
  pharynx, larynx, trachea,
  urethra.

Systemic absorption is not a serious risk provided local analgesic drugs are not applied to inflamed areas, and provided rules about dosage are remembered. Pressurized sprays deliver a metered amount of drug. They can be useful as a first stage in the nose or on the gums and are also used for laryngotracheal analgesia. Packs soaked with 4% lignocaine are commonly applied to the nose. The cornea is readily made insensitive by many local analgesic drugs but more than one application may be necessary. Repeated applications are necessary for conjunctival analgesia. Local analgesia of the urethra is very useful in the male but should not be performed if a connection is known to exist between the bulbous urethra and the corpus cavernosus since local anaesthetic can then enter the systemic circulation rapidly.

Intravenous regional analgesia

This is a most important and useful method of analgesia for limb surgery or manipulation. A volume of local analgesic drug is introduced into the venous system of an exsanguinated limb and kept therein by an arterial tourniquet. Analgesia results in about 5 minutes.

Ischaemia can, by itself, cause analgesia; the onset is then much slower than if an analgesic is added although the thicker motor fibres of nerves are affected first. Recovery from intravenous regional analgesia is slower than recovery from ischaemia. The analgesic agent diffuses peripherally and is fixed to nervous elements.

Large muscle masses of the leg make this method somewhat unsatisfactory in practice, but it is a common method in casualty departments for surgery on the arm.

Method. A small cannula is introduced into a vein in the limb to be operated upon, flushed free of blood and strapped firmly in place. The limb is then raised so as to drain all the blood from it. If the surgical condition will allow exsanguination can be made more complete by means of an Esmarch rubber bandage. This is applied tightly from the distal to the proximal part of the limb. A double pneumatic cuff is now applied around the proximal part of the limb including a pad of cotton wool to protect nerves. The upper cuffs is inflated to a pressure much higher than systolic arterial pressure. (The lower cuff is used later). The limb is then lowered, taking care that the cuff pressure is maintained.

A volume (20—30 ml) of local analgesic drug is then injected into the cannula. The identity and concentration of this drug must be carefully checked. This solution should *not* have adrenaline added to it. A common drug is 0.5% lignocaine, but 0.5% prilocaine is less toxic although the amount of methaemoglobin in the blood does rise after the cuff has been released. This is probably unimportant in fit adults, but may be hazardous if oxygen flux is already compromized by intercurrent pathology. Prilocaine causes fewer neurological symptoms and signs than lignocaine when the cuff is released. Lignocaine causes superficial analgesia but sometimes this is not sufficient for reduction of fractures, and prilocaine is now regarded as the drug of choice.

The volume of the solution injected depends on the location of the occluding cuff. This can be applied to the upper or lower part of a limb; less drug is required for a small volume of tissue. Maximum safe dosages should never be exceeded but care with the remainder of the manoeuvre adds to the safety of this technique. The occluding cuff should not be released within 20 minutes of injection since during this time the drug is being fixed to nervous tissue. The distal cuff (of the double cuffs) is now inflated to avoid pain from the more proximal cuff since the latter site is not affected by the local analgesic. Surgery can be performed as soon as analgesia is evident.

Estimation of general systemic plasma levels after release of the cuff suggests that about 50% of a dose is retained in the limb. In elderly patients the occluding cuff should be released and then reinflated to limit washout of the drug. Bilateral cuffs should never be released at the same time.

The general use of tourniquets suggests that 1½ hours should be the maximum period of use. Sensation reappears almost immediately after the cuff is released so alternative analgesia may be required quickly and the technique is, of course, inappropriate if haemostasis needs to be checked by release of the tourniquet before the operation is completed.

Historically, and in other countries, intravenous local analgesic drugs have also been employed as general anaesthetic agents. Lignocaine is commonly used in bolus doses as an antidysrhythmic drug.

Toxic effects of local analgesic drugs

In contrast to many other drugs it must be a rare event for a clinician to fail to observe the onset of toxic signs of local analgesics when they occur. However, it is unfortunately true that not all those who use these drugs know how to manage the complications. It is indefensible' for a doctor to inject a foreign substance and yet to be ignorant about potentially life-threatening results. These are not common but when they do occur it is frequently possible to observe that there has been a basic error in technique.

The symptoms and signs described below arise in two different ways:
  abnormal systemic absorption,
  peculiar patient sensitivity.
The latter is rare.

Abnormal systemic absorption results from:
  inadvertent intravenous injection,
  use of agent in inflamed or vascular tissue,
  use of large volumes of concentrated solutions,
  use of solutions without vasoconstrictors.

The *results of systemic absorption* are seen as symptoms and signs referable to the:
  central nervous,
  circulatory, and
  respiratory systems.

Feelings of unease, anxiety, peri-oral tingling and panic develop in some patients; others become euphoric. These symptoms may be followed by signs of *central* depression and convulsions.

Acute *cardiovascular* collapse is manifested by hypotension and bradycardia.

Respiratory failure occurs from central depression of the medulla and apnoea, or from central paralysis of the muscles of respiration.

Treatment. The cellular requirement is for oxygen. This may be achieved either by paralysis with muscle relaxants and controlled ventilation with oxygen or, in the less serious cases, with *modest* doses of intravenous thiopentone or diazepam to abort the convulsions. Intubation of the trachea is not an easy manoeuvre in a patient with convulsions but it may be essential to ensure patency of the airway if ventilation with a bag and mask is unsuccessful.

Cardiovascular collapse is treated with intravenous fluids which must be rapidly transfused. The legs may be raised at the hips to supply an immediate autotransfusion.

The importance of competence in the resuscitative manoeuvres outlined above is clear. This does not mean, however, that only anaesthetists can perform them. All medical staff could, and indeed should, be able to make a reasonable attempt at resuscitation.

The effects of abnormal systemic absorption depend on a number of variables:

 age,
 size,
 weight,
 nutritional state,
 general health,
 metabolism of local analgesic drug,
 prophylactic premedication.

To some extent at least, the development of systemic reactions to local analgesics is related to the *age* of the recipient. The amount of drug injected into an elderly patient should not only be based on body weight but also be adjusted for that patient's age. The effects of a systemic reaction in an elderly patient are more serious than in a fit young patient. For example, someone who is hypoxic at rest cannot tolerate an increase in methaemoglobinaemia from prilocaine, which in turn causes further reduction in the carriage of oxygen. Again, a patient with coronary insufficiency is seriously at risk if coronary perfusion is further impaired as a result of the direct depressant effect on myocardial contractility caused by lignocaine. An elderly patient who has cerebral atherosclerosis is less able to withstand the effects of convulsions.

Some local analgesic drugs whose linkage between the hydrophilic and lipophilic parts is by an amide are *metabolized* in the liver.

Examples of these are lignocaine, prilocaine and bupivacaine. Others whose linkage is by means of an ester (excluding cocaine) are hydrolysed by plasma cholinesterase. Procaine and 2-chloroprocaine are examples of these. It is clear that the latter group of drugs may be preferable in those patients peculiarly at risk from systemic reactions.

The role of *premedication* in the prevention of systemic reactions is important. Barbiturates and benzodiazepines are specifically indicated since both drugs raise the threshold and excitability of cortical neurones to stimulation and thus diminish the likelihood of convulsions.

Appropriate equipment must be both available and functional. Systemic reactions to local analgesics can be successfully managed and carry a good prognosis. The risk of their occurrence should not deter a well-trained doctor from the use of these techniques.

Spinal and epidural analgesia

The methods have points of similarity and of contrast. A needle is introduced between the spinous processes of two vertebrae and passed through the ligamentum flavum. In the case of a spinal (intradural) analgesic a fine needle is advanced until the subarachnoid space is identified by the escape of cerebrospinal fluid. In epidural analgesia a thicker needle is used and the subarachnoid space is not breached.

There are few, if any, *absolute indications* for the use of these techniques for surgical operations. There are several *relative* indications. They represent alternatives to full general anaesthesia, they can be supplemented by general anaesthesia and they can be used as analgesic techniques for mothers in labour or for patients with unremitting pain.

Each method has some disadvantages and advantages for surgical operations, but spinal analgesia is less often practised than epidural. There are reasons for this difference. On the one hand, there were a very few, ghastly, paralytic complications of spinal analgesia which occurred more than 30 years ago and on the other, there is the fact that epidural techniques have become well known because they are common in the current practice of obstetric departments. Modern technology has provided better equipment than was available hitherto, with the result that spinal analgesia is undoubtedly safer than it used to be but, notwithstanding, it is still used infrequently.

It is often stated that spinal or epidural techniques are useful for patients who have respiratory disability resulting from chronic pulmonary disease. It is mistakenly thought that these patients are so difficult to anaesthetize with a general anaesthetic that therefore a regional one is to be preferred.

Another error is to imagine that postoperative chest complications are less likely following spinal or epidural analgesia. General anaesthesia allows the opportunity for tracheal suction so that accumulated secretions can readily be removed during, or at the end, of an operation. This is not possible during regional analgesia.

The ability to cough is impaired irrespective of the anaesthetic technique. In the case of a patient under a general anaesthetic this is because of central and peripheral depression and depressed ciliary activity. In the case of a patient who has received regional analgesia the disability may arise because a deep breath prior to coughing is impossible. The patient has to lie still on the operating table during regional analgesia, and it is this which tends to lead to accumulation of bronchial secretions. There may, however, be some advantage in epidural techniques with an indwelling catheter so that postoperative pain relief may be provided, but this is not always relevant to the decision to use regional analgesia rather than general anaesthesia.

Absolute *contraindications* do exist to the use of these techniques for surgery. Active skin infection over the area of injection is an obvious one. The presence of neurological disease is another, because were there to be any deterioration postoperatively then the technique of analgesia would be blamed. Skeletal disease, deformity of the spine or ossification of spinal ligaments are further contraindications, although these may only be relative to the skill of the anaesthetist and the desirability of or the need for, the technique. The presence of a pre-existing bleeding diathesis, caused by disease or drugs, or the need for systemic anticoagulation during surgery are absolute contraindications to epidural analgesia because of the risk that a haematoma might follow inadvertent damage to a blood vessel and press on the spinal cord or nerve roots. Patients who habitually suffer from headaches should not have spinal analgesia unless no alternative exists; post-spinal headache (see later) is bound to occur.

Spinal analgesia involves the injection of, usually hyperbaric, solutions into the cerebrospinal fluid. The spread of analgesic solutions is determined by:

the dose
the site of injection,
the posture of the patient during and after the injection.

The latter can be easily adjusted once the desired level of analgesia has been achieved by an appropriate tilt of the table. Spinal analgesia for surgical purposes is usually established below L1 or 2 at which level the spinal cord ends in adults, thus the risk of direct damage is avoided.

This technique has the limitation that once the injection has been made there is no way of modifying the result unless an intradural catheter is used for supplementary doses of the drug. Continuous spinal analgesia is not now recommended because of the increased risk of infection or of physical damage to the spinal cord.

Epidural analgesia is probably more difficult as a technique than spinal analgesia because the end point depends on the observation of a change in resistance to pressure whereas, in most cases, a successful spinal puncture will be heralded by the appearance of cerebrospinal fluid at the hub of the needle. Thick needles are used for epidural analgesia so that these changes in resistance to the passage of the needle can be readily appreciated. Wide-bore needles allow catheters to be passed through their lumen into the epidural space.

There is a subatmospheric pressure in the epidural space which is at least partly caused by the tenting of the dural by the epidural needle. This may be detected by a variety of technical manoeuvres. After a small test dose of local analgesic to exclude inadvertent dry subarachnoid puncture a larger volume of solution is introduced through the needle or through the catheter which is passed into the epidural space. The extent of the analgesia which results depends mainly on the volume of the injection and only partly upon the posture of the patient. Extra solution can, of course be injected to supplement both the level of analgesia and its extent.

The lumbar approach is the common one but the epidural space can be entered at any level. *Caudal* analgesia is an approach at the lower end of the sacrum between the sacral cornua, but is otherwise no different from lumbar epidural analgesia.

Benefits of spinal or epidural analgesia

These techniques are enthusiastically proclaimed by some protagonists but other anaesthetists find little or no use for them.

Hypotension follows sympathetic paralysis, and vasodilatation can be very useful when the prevention of blood loss is important. Provided that it is possible to arrange the posture of the patient so that the field of operation is higher than the rest of the body, then relative ischaemia limits haemorrhage. Recovery from this hypotension is gradual so that reactionary bleeding tends not to occur.

Muscular relaxation is profound while the movements necessary for adequate ventilation need not be limited.

The bowel is contracted once the sympathetic supply is interrupted because vagal action is unopposed. This is a very useful benefit in pelvic or rectal surgery.

Patients with some *systemic disease,* for example, diabetes mellitus, myasthenia gravis or extreme obesity may have less disturbance in their therapy if they can be managed with these methods. Large muscular patients have less systemic disturbance after a regional than after a general anaesthetic.

Disadvantages of spinal or epidural analgesia

In addition to those already mentioned there are a number of limitations which affect all members of the operating team. The techniques are time-consuming; it is impossible to rush a regional technique and to do so invites failure. Staff in the operating room must be quiet; a noisy environment is not pleasant for the patient who may not understand the significance of what he hears. The patient may feel sensations of touch but suitable encouragement will usually allay anxiety. It is most important that this reassurance should be positive: patients under any form of local analgesic should be asked 'Are you quite comfortable?' and no suggestive questions about pain should ever be posed.

Post dural puncture headache occurs in about 15% of patients but it does not occur after an epidural anaesthetic. Headache also occurs after lumbar puncture. The incidence and severity are lessened now narrow gauge spinal needles are used, but accidental dural puncture during the course of an epidural with a large bore needle remains a cause of headache. The headache is unlike any other and is aggravated in the vertical posture. Most of the headaches are due to leakage of cerebrospinal fluid so that the brain is less well supported. Patients should be kept flat for 24 hours postoperatively and, if convenient, turned into the prone position. Oral fluids should be actively encouraged if possible, or failing that intravenous fluids should be given generously. This is to encourage replacement of cerebrospinal fluid by increased secretion in the choroid plexus. An epidural catheter can be introduced at another interspace and a continuous epidural infusion of Ringer lactate solution commenced. This has the effect also of raising the pressure in the epidural space and thus prevents further leakage of cerebrospinal fluid. The hole in the dura can be sealed by blood clot to prevent leakage of cerebrospinal fluid: 10 ml of the patient's blood is introduced in a sterile manner to the epidural space. The pain relief is often dramatic. Carbon dioxide inhalation can also reduce the headache; it is presumed that cerebral blood flow is increased and that thus secretion by the choroid plexus is increased. Mild analgesics should also be prescribed. The headache may last for several days and up to two weeks.

Meningeal infection is the most feared complication but it is very rare. Bacterial or chemical inflammation may occur and this may be followed by chronic inflammatory arachnoiditis. The end result may be paraplegia, paralysis or permanent weakness of the bladder sphincter or legs.

Backache occurs after both spinal and epidural techniques and is associated particularly with poor technique. A patient with a prolapsed intervertebral disc should probably not have epidural or spinal analgesia since mild trauma to the nerve roots is not uncommon. In addition any regression afterwards will, as with neurological disease, be blamed upon the analgesic method.

Sixth cranial nerve palsy can occur after general anaesthesia as well as after spinal analgesia. It is believed to be due to stretching of the nerve in its extradural course and it carries a good prognosis.

Continuous epidural analgesia

This is a most useful way of helping patients to cope with postoperative pain, particularly abdominal pain. At least part of the ventilatory defect during the postoperative period is due to diaphragmatic and abdominal muscle rigidity. A patient who is in pain tends to breathe very rapidly and shallowly. The occasional vital capacity breath is not taken. If this pain is abolished the patient can breathe quietly and regularly: deep breaths are possible when they are required.

It is impossible to cough effectively without taking a deep breath. Coughing and vigorous physiotherapy are possible after effective analgesia. (There are naturally other ways to achieve this desirable end-point which are not relevant here (see page 63); they include intravenous analgesics combined with non-specific respiratory stimulants, intercostal nerve blocks and self-administered analgesics or inhalation of low concentrations of nitrous oxide, methoxyflurane or trichlorethylene.)

The epidural catheter should ideally be placed near the median segment which needs to be blocked. Small volumes of analgesic solution can then be injected, and the hypotension which may follow any spread to higher segments can thus be avoided.

Bupivacaine, 0.25% or 0.125%, is again the drug of choice; the addition of adrenaline is not required since the drug is effective for 4–6 hours or even longer on occasions. The epidural catheter is strapped over the patient's shoulder and closed by a bacterial filter. Injections must be prepared carefully and are usually given by a doctor. The blood pressure must be checked and recorded frequently for 20 minutes after injection, because of the risks of hypotension from sympathetic paralysis.

7. Applied physiology in anaesthesia and intensive care

The state of anaesthesia is complex. It is hardly a normal condition, and thus to affirm that there are some lessons in physiology to be learnt from its study may appear at first sight to be somewhat contradictory. Just as the response to surgery interferes with the anticipated pharmacological action of drugs (see Chapter 4), so both anaesthesia and surgery may interfere with normal physiological responses. It is, however, certainly true that some physiological responses may be exemplified by an anaesthetized patient and furthermore that some of the phenomena of the anaesthetic state itself can only be understood by appreciating some physiology.

Changes occur in the normal physiological function of all systems as a result of anaesthesia. These, in turn, may require therapeutic intervention which itself may have effects on function. Disease processes similarly have effects which may also be mitigated by therapy.

This chapter is concerned with all of these, inextricably interwoven, aspects. The cardiovascular and respiratory systems are considered in some detail, since not only are they often causative of the changes in other systems, but also they are the two which are most obviously concerned in the moment-to-moment welfare of patients.

Cardiovascular system

The actions of anaesthetic drugs on normal physiological function throughout the body are mostly depressant. Cardiovascular function is no different in this respect from any other. This is somewhat mitigated by the stimulatory effect of increased activity of the sympathetic autonomic nervous system which occurs in response to several agents. The overall changes roughly parallel the relative potency and dose of the individual agents. Further modification can result from intercurrent changes in blood gas tensions and surgical stimulation.

Cardiovascular effects of general anaesthesia

The following account refers mainly to the effects of halothane.

Venodilatation is caused by relaxation of vascular smooth muscle: this happens early in anaesthesia and is followed later by arteriolar dilatation. If anaesthesia were to be induced in a patient whose venous return was dependent upon widespread vasoconstriction, for example, cardiac failure or after haemorrhage, it is probable that this vasodilatation would cause a precipitate decrease in venous return and thus in cardiac output. In normal, healthy persons, large doses of intravenous thiopentone can tend to cause the same effect, although the increase in the adrenal output of catecholamines (which is not prevented by thiopentone) usually results in tachycardia.

Baroreceptor activity occurs in the conscious state during hypertension, and stimulates central reflexes to lower the blood pressure by bradycardia and by vasodilatation. The frequency of baroreceptor afferent discharge is increased although the threshold to stimulation, the central integrative processes and the efferent activity are all depressed as a result of anaesthesia. Bradycardia is a particular feature of halothane anaesthesia.

The myocardium itself is directly depressed so that contractility is impaired. Ganglionic blockade, alpha-receptor blockade and beta-receptor stimulation all increase dilatation in a variety of sites of the peripheral circulation during halothane anaesthesia.

These mechanisms combine to produce general depression of the cardiovascular system. Cardiac output is reduced by many of the above effects and, in addition, by independent diminution of venous return. This is caused by the reduced amplitude of excursion of the diaphragm and skeletal muscle relaxation, both of which contribute, in the conscious subject, to the maintenance of venous return. Catastrophic impairment of venous return can occur if the inferior vena cava is compressed by a gravid uterus: patients who are in the last trimester of pregnancy are placed supine with a wedge under their right side to allow the uterus to fall away from the inferior vena cava not only when general anaesthesia is induced, but also whenever they are recumbent.

The reduction in cardiac output on induction, usually not more than 30%, is not out of proportion to the reduction in the requirement for oxygen by the body. On some occasions, however, the reduction may be greater and hypoxia in some tissues may occur.

Mode of ventilation

Inappropriately *high inflation pressures* applied during controlled ventilation may cause a reduction in cardiac output as a result of direct pressure upon the heart which is transmitted from the lungs (cf. cardiac tamponade). The application of a resistance to expiration, or a fixed pressure against which the patient must exhale, may also have the same effect. If compensatory vasoconstriction is possible then cardiac output is maintained.

When a patient breathes halothane spontaneously a degree of *respiratory acidosis* develops to the extent that the arterial carbon dioxide tension may be as much as 8.0 kPa (60 mmHg). This is not apparently harmful for it happens in many operating rooms without disaster. Most other inhaled anaesthetic agents reduce the output of catecholamines but halothane does not. When hypercapnia develops during halothane anaesthesia the customary increase in catecholamines still occurs and may be responsible for the absence of harm. When, however, a patient receives controlled ventilation it is particularly important to remember that *hyperventilation* reduces cardiac output (see Chapter 5). This dependence of cardiac output upon arterial carbon dioxide tension during anaesthesia is such that there may be as much as 0.75 litre/min change in cardiac output if the arterial carbon dioxide tension changes 2.6 kPa (20 mmHg) in either direction from the normal of around 5.3 kPa (40 mmHg).

Dysrhythmias

Some anaesthetic agents sensitize the heart so that ventricular dysrhythmias occur more readily. The effect is made significantly worse by the simultaneous occurrence of hypoxia, hypercapnia or overdose of the agent. The importance of a dysrhythmia is that haemodynamics may be affected, so that cardiac output and coronary perfusion are reduced and myocardial hypoxia results. This may precipitate further dysrhythmias and even ventricular fibrillation.

If a patient is inadequately anaesthetized for the surgical procedure one of two responses may occur both of which are abolished by an increase in the depth of anaesthesia. The commoner is sympathetic stimulation which results in tachycardia and hypertension. When the stimulus arises, traction on the peritoneum around the coeliac plexus or gall bladder or from the pleura around the pulmonary hilum, the other response occurs which is bradycardia and hypotension. It is due either to decreased sympathetic or increased parasympathetic activity.

Acute blood loss

Diagnosis

Sudden dramatic haemorrhage may occur at any instant and without warning. The surgical incident which causes it may be anticipated or it may be accidental. Sometimes haemorrhage of a modest amount of blood has an effect out of all proportion to its size because it has been preceded by slow and continuous bleeding. Inspection of the anaesthetic chart (Fig. 5.19) may be informative in these cases. Patients with widespread arteriosclerotic disease may also react excessively to small losses.

The signs of haemorrhage under general anaesthesia are those one would expect:

    pallor,
    tachycardia,
    central venous hypotension,
    arterial hypotension, and
    oliguria.

Compensatory vasoconstriction in muscle and skin blood vessels may neither be so prompt nor so intense during anaesthesia as when the subject is conscious. This is particularly so when regional analgesia has paralysed the sympathetic outflow from the spinal cord. Compensatory tachycardia may not produce an increase in cardiac output because depression of myocardial contractility limits the strength of contraction.

Students may have seen recordings of the response of other animals to haemorrhage. Intact man is seldom monitored prior to haemorrhage unless this happens during a surgical operation. Vasoconstriction and hypotension occur after haemorrhage. The changes of vasoconstriction may be obscured under anaesthesia but they may be observed occasionally. The early response to haemorrhage is manifest by pallor and an increase in systolic arterial blood pressure, but the central venous pressure declines. This is soon followed by a fall in systolic arterial blood pressure and a continued, low central venous pressure (see Fig 5.19).

Treatment

The blood volume of an adult is 70 ml/kg, that of a neonate 80 ml/kg and that of an adult woman 65 ml/kg. In the absence of pre-existing anaemia a patient can lose 10% (i.e. 500 ml in an adult) without transfusion of blood. Blood substitutes are used whenever it is reasonable to anticipate that the total blood loss will not exceed 1000 ml; such forecasts are not always possible.

Blood transfusion is naturally the treatment of choice. The volume of blood lost is not always measured precisely and estimates of the volume required for transfusions have to be made. It is therefore useful to monitor blood replacement; serial measurements of the two vascular pressures are again required (see Chapter 5). If the loss is rapid there is no virtue in delay before blood is replaced and rapid transfusion is required.

Blood transfusion. Transfused blood must be warmed to 37°C because cold blood transfusion encourages serious dysrhythmias and, if large volumes are administered, hypothermia. In addition, cold causes venoconstriction and this slows the rate of transfusion. The filtration of micro aggregates (greater than 40 μm) which accumulate in blood older than 5 days seems a reasonable precaution despite lack of evidence that filtration in the pulmonary capillaries does harm. Very large transfusions may necessitate correction of the induced metabolic acidosis, hyperkalaemia and hypocalcaemia which follow transfusion. These are rarely serious enough to warrant treatment as a routine because dilution in the remaining blood volume is usually sufficient to offset their effects. Transfused blood is dangerous material. It is neither immediately as efficient in oxygen carriage, nor as efficient in thrombogenesis, as is unshed blood and for this reason, if for no other, crystalloid or colloid solutions are often substituted.

Other fluids. Occasionally cross-matched blood may not be available, and volumetric replacement with colloid solutions, which remain in the vascular compartment for varying periods, may have to be used. There are a number of possible preparations:

> Dextran 70,
> gelatin,
> hydroxyethyl starch,
> reconstituted plasma,
> plasma protein fraction, and
> albumin.

Each of these has advantages and disadvantages but none yet can be used to replace blood completely.

The usefulness of *central venous monitoring* during anaesthesia has led to its somewhat uncritical use in intensive therapy units. It is important to understand that the central venous pressure is representative solely of the filling pressure of the *right* heart. If the right ventricle cannot deal with an increased load then the central venous pressure rises. However, if the right heart does respond, and its stroke volume increases, then that increase in output is delivered to the left heart. The ability of the left side to respond is in turn indicated by left atrial pressure, but if this rises too rapidly pulmonary oedema may develop. This disaster may follow in spite of a normal central venous pressure. *The level of central venous pressure is not related to the development of pulmonary oedema.*

The *left atrial pressure* can be assessed indirectly by the determination of the pressure in the pulmonary artery. A balloon catheter is floated via a large vein through the right atrium and ventricle into the pulmonary artery. The pressure recorded when the catheter can be advanced no further is the wedge pressure. Pressure transducers and amplification systems are essential for this technique which, although expensive, is becoming more widely used. The catheter used for this pressure measurement is often combined with one other, and a thermistor is incorporated at its tip so that cardiac (left) output can be determined by thermal dilution. The latter technique involves the injection of small (10 ml) volumes of saline, of known temperature, into the right atrium and the detection of the consequent changes of temperature in the pulmonary arterial blood by means of the thermistor. The shape of the curve of change of temperature is related to cardiac output.

Respiratory system

There are several changes in respiratory function which accompany anaesthesia. Probably the commonest and most obvious is *respiratory depression*. This is manifest as a reduced minute volume of ventilation, either as a result of a reduction in the frequency of breathing or in the volume of each breath. Fig. 7.1 shows how a narcotic diminishes the sensitivity of the respiratory centre to inhaled carbon dioxide. Similar depression occurs in response to inhaled drugs. Close observation of the movement of the reservoir bag (see Chapter 3) is the most basic of all the methods in everyday practice, but more objective and more esoteric methods are becoming widely employed. Some methods of monitoring ventilation are described in Chapter 5, and the importance of efficient carbon dioxide elimination is there explained.

If, or when, cardiac output decreases, pulmonary blood flow must also decrease. Some alveoli then receive less blood and therefore gas

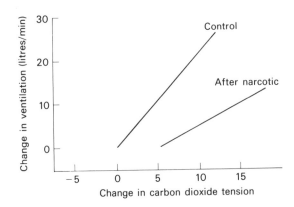

Fig. 7.1. Idealized carbon dioxide response curve. Note shift of zero and change of slope.

exchange is impaired. This is, as it were, a waste of ventilation and can be quantified as an increase in *physiological dead space*. If there were no respiratory compensation, which there is, an increase in arterial carbon dioxide tension would be inevitable.

When a subject lies down the diaphragm rises: this reduces the volume left in the lungs at the end of a normal expiration. Thus, this volume, known as the *functional residual capacity*, is reduced. There is a further reduction on induction of anaesthesia. Abdominal distension aggravates the effect. One of the functions of the functional residual capacity is to minimize the effects of changes in concentration of inspired gases: it acts as a buffer. Partly as a consequence of its reduction there is a decrease in the distensibility of the lungs, that is to say, a decrease in *compliance* (compliance is defined as volume change per unit change of applied pressure). The lungs become a little stiffer. This increase in stiffness can be temporarily reversed by a deep breath but, within 5 minutes, the lung compliance is again as low as it was before.

The most important result, however, of this reduction in lung volume is the effect it has on the *venous admixture*. Not all of the cardiac output passes through functional parts of the lung: some is bypassed through anatomical channels and some perfuses alveoli which are not simultaneously ventilated. The sum of these two fractions is expressed as a percentage of cardiac output and is called the venous admixture. It is the perfusion equivalent of physiological dead space; that is to say, it is wasted perfusion. The proportion of wasted perfusion increases during anaesthesia.

Normally, ventilation is matched to blood flow so that the ratio between the two, called the *ventilation: perfusion ratio*, ($\dot{V}_A : \dot{Q}$), for both lungs is about 0.8. The distribution of both gas and blood is determined partly by the forces of gravity which act on the thorax. Apical blood flow, for example, is less than that to the bases of the lungs when the subject is erect. However, when the subject is lain down this relationship is different and the matching between ventilation and blood flow is disturbed. Both the respiratory depression and the decrease in cardiac output of anaesthesia also affect the ratio. Very sophisticated direct measurements have demonstrated that the $\dot{V}_A : \dot{Q}$ is altered by the induction of anaesthesia and that the changes are similar to those of some chronic respiratory disease. (The frequency distribution of the ratios is broadened.) It is clear that mismatching contributes to the venous admixture effect described above.

The potentially deleterious effects of anaesthesia on oxygenation and carbon dioxide homeostasis are minimized, but not eliminated by, two manoeuvres. Firstly, most anaesthetists use at least 30% oxygen in the inspired mixture, and secondly, many patients receive controlled ventilation of their lungs.

One of the effects of increased inspired oxygen concentration is that concomitant hypoventilation in a spontaneously breathing patient may be masked. The clinical appearance of the patient remains satisfactory but alveolar ventilation may be so reduced that the arterial carbon dioxide tensions may increase to high, not to say dangerous, levels (see Chapter 5). Another effect may be that cardiac output increases as a result of improved oxygenation.

Effects of controlled ventilation

Controlled ventilation is frequently necessary during a general anaesthetic or during intensive therapy but like any other treatment, it has disadvantages as well as advantages. The reduction in functional residual capacity which occurs as a result of induction of anaesthesia is less if ventilation is controlled. There is immediate compensation for alveolar hypoventilation although some forms of controlled ventilation may themselves cause an increase in physiological dead space. The distribution of inspired gases may be different and, when inspiratory flow rates are needlessly high, preferential distribution may occur to

areas of the lung which do not have appropriate perfusion. Oxygenation
may not always therefore be improved.

Controlled ventilation differs from spontaneous ventilation. Fig. 7.2
shows one aspect of the difference on which all the other effects depend.
The intrapleural pressure changes are important. The diaphragm
moves downwards and the chest wall moves outwards during the inspiratory phase of spontaneous ventilation. This results in the parietal
pleura moving similarly and thus the extant subatmospheric pressure in
the intrapleural space becomes more subatmospheric. The elastic lung
consequently expands and air is drawn in. The reverse happens in
expiration.

When controlled ventilation is imposed opposite pressure changes
take place. The intrapleural pressure reaches a (positive) peak at the end
of inspiration and returns usually to atmospheric, or slightly subatmospheric, pressure at the end of expiration.

The existence of a subatmospheric intrapleural pressure during spontaneous ventilation has important effects on blood flow in the vena cava.
This flow is increased during inspiration — the *thoracic pump mechanism*. Abolition of this effect during controlled ventilation contributes
to the decreased cardiac output because venous return is thereby reduced.
The central venous pressure is apparently increased during controlled
ventilation but this does not necessarily indicate a change in right ven-

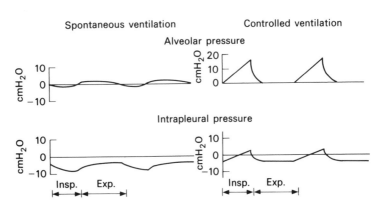

Fig. 7.2. Comparison of the alveolar and intrapleural pressures during spon-
taneous and controlled ventilation. From Mushin W.W., Rendell-Baker L.,
Thompson P.W. & Mapleson W.W. (1969) *Automatic Ventilation of the Lungs,*
Blackwell Scientific Publications, Oxford, with permission

tricular function and is only a reflection of increased intrathoracic pressure.

The direct effect (cardiac tamponade) of intrathoracic pressure upon cardiac output has been mentioned above and in addition, the pulmonary alveolar capillaries are exposed to the effects of the raised intrathoracic pressure. Lobar pulmonary blood flow is decreased during the inspiratory phase of controlled ventilation.

The benefits of controlled ventilation in most clinical circumstances outweigh any harmful effects it may have.

Controlled ventilation may be applied by two means:

> manual ventilation,
> automatic ventilators.

Manual ventilation is seldom used except as a temporary expedient (see Chapter 8); automatic ventilation with one of the bewildering variety of machines (see Chapter 3) is commonly employed.

It is essential for the safe practice of this technique that there is always an alternative means of ventilation available at the bedside (e.g. a self-filling bag). Failures of machines are not uncommon and this is a minimum requirement. It is obvious also that there must be trained personnel to supervise the patient.

Effects of raised airway pressure during expiration

Hypoxaemia which results from decreased functional residual capacity is reduced, if not abolished, by the maintenance of a positive pressure in the airway. This can be arranged during spontaneous or controlled ventilation. The addition of a positive pressure in expiration requires that peak inspiratory pressure must also be raised to avoid a resultant decrease in ventilation. The combined effect of both these manoeuvres is that cardiac output is reduced and there is a real risk of pneumothorax. Oligaemia in the pulmonary vascular system may result in an increased secretion of antidiuretic hormone and fluid retention. There is also decreased venous flow in the pelvis and legs with the consequent increased risk of venous thrombosis.

Postoperative hypoxaemia

There is a reduction in the arterial oxygen tension in postoperative patients after general anaesthesia. This has been demonstrated after anaesthesia has lasted more than 20 minutes and in patients older than

12 years. It is by no means clear why it occurs, but again it is believed to be due to the decrease in functional residual capacity which is not reversed immediately at the end of an operation. The demand for oxygen increases postoperatively when the patient begins to awaken, perhaps in pain, and particularly when postoperative shivering occurs. The response to loss of heat, which occurs as a result of the widespread vasodilatation of general anaesthesia, is firstly increased muscle tone and secondly overt shivering. The cardiac output may still be reduced, and/or the blood volume may also be less than normal, so that oxygen extraction of the tissues has to be increased. Mixed venous blood has therefore a lower oxygen tension than usual and this contributes to the lower arterial oxygen tension. Ventilatory impairment is not a feature of postoperative hypoxaemia: arterial carbon dioxide tension is usually normal.

Deep breathing is encouraged and oxygen is provided to counteract the hypoxaemia (see Chapter 3). Elderly patients should receive oxygen enriched air for at least 24 hours postoperatively, because for them hypoxaemia lasts longer.

Respiratory failure

The management of that degree of deterioration in respiratory function which occurs during general anaesthesia has already been described in outline, but patients with respiratory failure are also found in general wards and in intensive therapy units. Similar features exist which help in the appreciation of the disordered function.

Progressive deterioration of respiratory function has been classified as:

respiratory impairment,
respiratory inadequacy,
respiratory failure.

These terms are the preferred ones; chronic respiratory failure is a descriptive phrase which encompasses the last two states but also includes a degree of metabolic compensation for respiratory acidosis.

Respiratory failure may be:

absolute, or
relative.

Absolute respiratory failure exists during:

apnoea, or
asphyxiation.

Relative respiratory failure may be due to:

hypoventilation, or

failure of oxygenation, combined with normo- or hyper-ventilation.

Table 7.1 summarizes some examples of these types of respiratory failure. It is clear, however, that as with many classifications which are designed to help this one fails because some disease processes or events fall simultaneously into more than one group. For example, a grossly obese patient with a head injury may be resuscitated from a temporary period of apnoea, inhale some stomach contents and, after momentary asphyxiation, develop pulmonary oedema. The final state of this hypothetical victim of circumstance is a combination of ventilatory and oxygenation failure. This is an extreme example but it does demonstrate the degree of complexity of the problems which are common in intensive therapy units.

Clinical diagnosis

The diagnosis of respiratory failure is a clinical one which may be substantiated by a few tests. It is important to understand that the tests merely demonstrate the extent of failure: they neither provide the diagnosis nor eliminate the need for proper clinical evaluation.

The *clinical signs* of respiratory failure are found in three systems.

Anxiety and restlessness, followed by unconsciousness and coma, are those arising from the *central nervous system*.

The *cardiovascular system* is also first stimulated and then depressed. Tachycardia, peripheral vasodilatation and hypertension are followed by hypotension, pallor and vasoconstriction.

Signs of failure in the *respiratory system* are firstly, an increase in ventilatory effort, and secondly, fatigue leading to physical exhaustion. The increase in effort is seen as dyspnoea and the use of the accessory muscles of respiration (sternomastoid, platysma); the presence of movements of accessory muscles uncoordinated with those of the diaphragm may result in the (non-pathognomic) sign of tracheal tug. Sweating, vasodilatation, hypertension and tachycardia are often referred to as signs of carbon dioxide accumulation, and certainly the lobster-red facies is descriptive of some patients with this condition. If it is unrelieved, the patient makes greater and greater respiratory efforts which gradually become irregular and finally the patient becomes unrousable, cyanosed and apnoeic.

Table 7.1 Examples of respiratory failure in the practice of anaesthesia

Type	Observation	Examples from general medicine	Examples from routine practice of general anaesthesia	
Absolute	Apnoea	No breathing	Cerebrovascular incident	Administration of muscle relaxant drugs
	Asphyxia	Total airway obstruction	Head injury Inhaled foreign body Acute epiglottitis Drowning	Unsupported jaw of unconscious patient
Relative	Ventilatory	Hypoventilation	Myasthenia gravis Polyneuritis Extreme obesity	Partial reversal of or recovery from muscle relaxants Respiratory depression following narcotics
	Oxygenation	Normo-/hyper-ventilation Hypoxia	Status asthmaticus Pulmonary oedema	Postoperative hypoxaemia

Confirmatory tests

Blood gas analysis of arterial blood is the most helpful, but the most abused, test in this field. It is as important when using this test, as with any other test performed in a laboratory, to ask two questions.

Can the result be interpreted?
Will the result affect my management of the patient?

These questions must be asked because there is a potential, perhaps not very great, risk to the patient owing to the method of sampling. Arterial puncture must be done properly and provided that it is, then this risk is acceptable.

The first question can only be answered affirmatively *if the inspired oxygen concentration is known.* If the patient is breathing an uncontrolled concentration of oxygen (MC mask, nasal oxygen etc.) it is negligent to risk damage to an artery and to waste the time of laboratory technicians in performing an analysis whose results cannot be properly interpreted. Air, if safe for the patient, or a known concentration of oxygen (high air flow oxygen enriched or 100% oxygen with a reservoir bag), should be administered for 10 minutes before the sample is taken; that concentration is recorded.

Interpretation is assisted by determining the 'virtual' shunt from the graph shown in Fig. 7.3. This diagram is used as follows. Suppose a patient is receiving 50% oxygen and the arterial oxygen tension is found to be 23 kPa (175 mmHg). Point A on the graph indicates that the patient has an approximate shunt of 8%. A lower concentration of oxygen could be prescribed without reducing the arterial oxygen tension to a dangerous extent — for example, point B.

It is common experience that patients cannot be successfully weaned from automatic ventilators unless the figure for virtual shunt is less than 10%. Notice that haemoglobin, cardiac output and ventilation must be approximately normal for this form of the relationship between inspired oxygen and arterial oxygen tension to be valid.

An answer to the second question is now possible.

One of the many decisions about the management of respiratory failure concerns the institution of controlled ventilation. This decision is seldom, if ever, made solely on the basis of arterial blood gas tensions, but is determined also by the history and physical signs. Other decisions concerned with the efficacy of therapy or the evolution of the disease

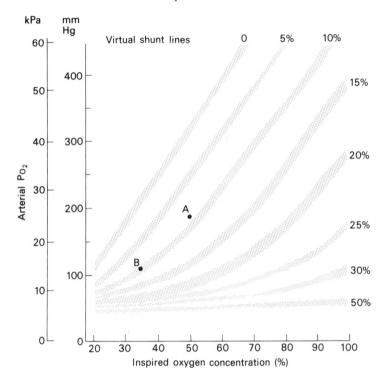

Fig. 7.3. Virtual shunt graph. Hb: 10–14 g/100 ml; Paco$_2$: 3.3–3.5 kPa (25–40 mmHg); a–vO$_2$ content diff.: 5 ml/100 ml. From Nunn J. F. (1978) *Applied Respiratory Physiology*, 2nd Edn. Butterworths, with permission.

process can only be made on the basis of serial arterial blood gas analyses and then these tests are invaluable and the answer to the second question is yes.

Reference values for arterial blood gas tensions are given in the Appendix. Respiratory failure is sometimes defined in terms of blood gas analysis results but, as has already been emphasised, this definition must not be made the sole basis for the diagnosis.

The *arterial carbon dioxide* tension is increased in respiratory failure. The extent to which ventilatory inefficiency or failure exists is demonstrated by the extent of the rise in the arterial carbon dioxide tension (see Chapter 5).

Some patients with chronic bronchitis and emphysema have arterial carbon dioxide tensions of about 6.5 kPa (50 mmHg) and are at work normally. Most clinicians would accept that respiratory failure exists if the value exceeds 7.3 kPa (55 mmHg) when the patient breathes air.

The *arterial oxygen tension* is decreased in respiratory failure. The extent of the decrease indicates the degree of failure of oxygenation. There are no compensatory mechanisms available to minimize the effects of such a decrease when it occurs acutely. Ventilation does increase but the uptake of oxygen in the pulmonary capillaries cannot be increased more than by a very small fraction by this response. The hazards of a decrease in arterial oxygen tension are serious although a tension of 9.2 kPa (70 mmHg) still results in a haemoglobin oxygen saturation of over 90%. If the arterial oxygen tension is less than 7.3 kPa (55 mmHg), and the patient is breathing air, again most clinicians would accept that respiratory failure is present. In chronic hypoxaemia, not only is ventilation increased, but cardiac output and red cell mass are also increased in the attempt to improve oxygen delivery to the tissues.

Measurement of the volumes of expired gas are also valuable but are sometimes misapplied. The serial measurement of *vital capacity* (the maximal expired volume after a maximal inspiration) is useful in detecting the progress (or regress) of respiratory muscle weakness in, for example myasthenia gravis. The ability to take a deep breath when it is required is an important indicator of ventilatory reserve. The function of this deep breath is probably associated with:

  prevention of collapse of alveoli,
  movement of particulate inhaled foreign matter and mucus,
  renewal of the surfactant lining of alveoli,
  the replenishment of the functional residual capacity with fresh air.

It is this last function which is important in incipient respiratory failure. When the respiratory centre senses an increase in hydrogen ions in the cerebrospinal fluid (caused by an increase in arterial carbon dioxide tension) a deep breath is signalled. If the muscles of respiration cannot respond, either by an increase in the tidal excursion, a deep breath or by an increase in respiratory frequency, there is no reserve. This absence of reserve is followed very rapidly by acute ventilatory failure. Arterial carbon dioxide tensions remain within the reference range until this point is reached. Once vital capacity breaths become impossible a rapid deterioration in carbon dioxide homeostasis occurs. Carbon dioxide narcosis is inevitable in the absence of therapy, and may be followed by cardiac arrest caused by hypoxia. One still unfortunately hears the plea, 'only a few hours ago the blood gas analysis was "normal" '; this indicates the above elementary lesson has not yet been learnt.

It is usually said that vital capacity should be twice tidal volume. Serial measurements of the latter may sometimes be sensitive enough to reveal the same progress, but because an effort is required and motivation is beneficial, vital capacity measurements are preferred.

Management of respiratory failure

This depends on the cause, the natural history of the disease and the degree of malfunction. Hypoventilation must be corrected, possibly with controlled ventilation. Hypoxia must be abolished as soon as possible, either by controlled oxygen therapy or by controlled ventilation with oxygen-enriched air. In patients with severe respiratory impairment spontaneous ventilation may be maintained by the *hypoxic* drive. The respiratory centre is no longer sensitive to changes in carbon dioxide tension. Abolition of hypoxaemia with uncontrolled oxygen therapy is dangerous since further rises in arterial carbon dioxide tension and apnoea may follow. The effect of controlled oxygen therapy with very low inspired concentrations (24%) of oxygen should be tested before any further increase in inspired oxygen is allowed. Respiratory depression caused by overdose of narcotic drugs can be treated with specific antagonists, and that caused by chronic hypercapnia or hypoxaemia can sometimes be reduced with central stimulants (analeptics). Muscle weakness may be corrected by anticholinesterase drugs. Severe lower airways obstruction may be reversed with bronchodilators which are best given intravenously rather than in aerosol form. Bacterial infection must be treated with appropriate antibiotics. Fluid retention may require aggressive diuretic therapy. Foreign bodies in the respiratory tract need to be removed by bronchoscopy. Physiotherapy is useful to encourage the removal of retained sputum. Temporary guarantee of the patency of the upper airway is achieved by nasotracheal intubation. Bulbar paresis may require that a tracheostomy be fashioned so that the lungs can be protected from aspiration.

Fluid balance system

It is customary to withhold fluids from patients for at least 6 hours before elective surgery. In practice, this period often amounts to as much as 12 hours because fluid administration is stopped arbitrarily at midnight. Thus, otherwise normal adult patients may come to operation with a fluid deficit of about 1000ml or even more. When dry, cold anaesthetic gases are inhaled there is a substantial usage of water in the process of humidification. Evaporation of sweat from the skin and evaporation of fluid from open cavities contribute to the cumulative fluid deficit. Oedema formation in the tissues after surgical procedure (and translocation of fluid, which occurs after trauma if not after surgery) may also result in fluid loss.

In the first 24–48 hours after operation there is fluid retention, and sodium retention lasts longer. Potassium excretion is increased postoperatively. These postoperative changes occur despite adequate fluid therapy, and they are believed to be due to increased secretion of antidiuretic hormone and increased secretion of adrenocortical hormones, particularly glucocorticoids.

Management. When a surgical operation and the necessary anaesthetic are likely to result in any delay before normal fluid intake resumes, it is both humane and sound therapy to provide some parenteral fluid. Replacement is usually with Hartmann's solution which contains the closest concentration of electrolytes to extracellular fluid. Isotonic saline (0.9%) and dextrose (5%) are sometimes given as alternatives. At least 500 ml is given in the first hour of surgery and thereafter about 250 ml per hour. Dextran 70 in saline or dextrose is a prophylactic against deep venous thrombosis and this is substituted for crystalloid solutions in some centres.

Urine output can be monitored during prolonged surgery. The effects of hypotension, which reduces urine output, can be clearly demonstrated. Sometimes it can be anticipated that renal blood flow is likely to be jeopardized or that urinary flow has ceased, and diuretics (frusemide or the osmotic diuretic, mannitol) may be given. Postoperatively, 30 ml urine per hour is regarded as satisfactory.

8. Techniques associated with resuscitation*

The term resuscitation may be used in different ways. These are:
resuscitation of the apparently dead,
resuscitation of the newborn, and
resuscitation of an unfit person prior to emergency surgery.

Resuscitation of the apparently dead includes respiratory resuscitation, which may be sufficient to prevent a terminal event, and it commonly has to be combined with cardiac resuscitation. Resuscitation of the newborn is merely one specialist application of general methods appropriately modified for special circumstances. Resuscitation of an unfit patient prior to surgery is particularly concerned with replenishment of blood volume following acute illness or injury.

Resuscitation of the apparently dead

Respiratory resuscitation

The differential diagnosis between apnoea and airway obstruction has already been discussed in Chapter 5, and will not be repeated here. Obstruction of the airway must be corrected urgently and, in any case, clarity of the airway is vital for successful performance of proper resuscitation.

Historical methods of respiratory resuscitation (Marshall Hall, Silvester, Schäfer, Holger Nielsen and Eve) rely on the assumption that the airway is clear. Expansion of the chest is caused by indirect means: gas enters the lungs provided that there is an unimpeded route for it. In the last 30 years or so, expired air resuscitation has become the method of choice and has been popularized to the extent that it has superseded all others.

---

* This is the only chapter in this book in which the student is encouraged to learn to *do* various manoeuvres. Manikins are widely available on which crude skills may be acquired, but they are no substitute for practical clinical experience.

128

Technique of expired-air resuscitation (see Fig. 8.1)

1 The victim is usually supine. However, this is by no means essential and the method has been used in the water or wherever an incident has occurred.
2 The airway must be cleared of vomit, foreign bodies, dentures or blood. The lower jaw may need elevation in order to keep the tongue away from the posterior pharyngeal wall.
3 The alternative airway must be closed, (i.e. the nostrils pinched if the mouth is to be used or the lips, if the nose is to be used).
4 The rescuer takes a deep breath and applies his mouth to that of the victim.
5 The rescuer blows his expired breath into the lungs of the victim and watches the chest rise and, after removal of his mouth, fall again.

This procedure should be performed about 12 times each minute.

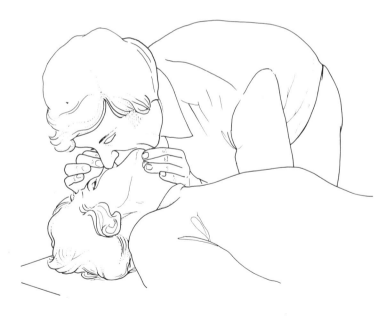

Fig. 8.1a   Expired-air resuscitation — inflation.

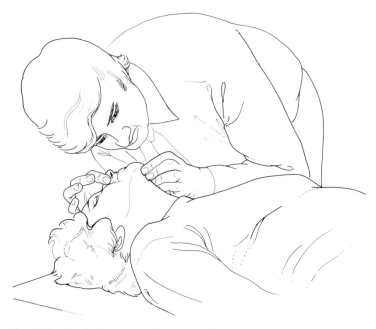

Fig. 8.1b   Expired-air resuscitation — exhalation.

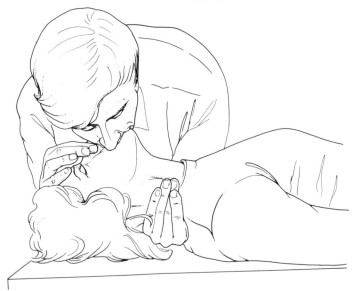

Fig. 8.1c   Expired-air resuscitation — alternative position of the left hand.

Why does expired-air resuscitation work?

The first part of an expired tidal volume contains the same concentration of oxygen as that at the end of the previous inspiration. This gas comes from the anatomical dead space of the rescuer and is about 150 ml in volume. The next part of the rescuer's expiration, which is greater than normal volume, obviously contains a lower concentration of oxygen than that inspired but it is not usually less than 15%. When the rescuer is breathing normal atmospheric air the combination of dead space gas (21% oxygen) and the increased volume of ventilation is sufficient to provide oxygen to and eliminate carbon dioxide from, the victim. Indeed, arterial blood gas analysis of blood from apnoeic and intubated patients during expired-air resuscitation shows that normal gas tensions can be maintained by this method.

Apparatus for respiratory resuscitation

One of the essential prerequisites for any rescue operation is that the need for equipment should be kept minimal. This is the case with expired-air resuscitation: in its simplest form none is needed. Fig. 8.2 a–d shows some simple means whereby the aesthetically unpleasant aspects of the technique may be reduced both conveniently and cheaply.

When the initial phase of resuscitation has been successfully achieved, ventilation is continued with a self-filling bag and mask. Fig. 8.3 shows how these devices work. One example is usually found in conventional packs of equipment for resuscitation in first aid posts, ambulances, general practice surgeries, casualty departments and hospital wards.

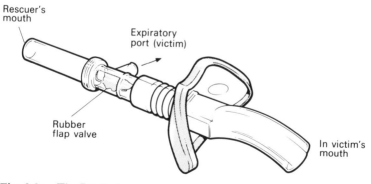

Fig. 8.2a   The Brook airway.

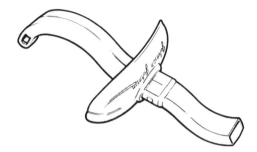

Fig. 8.2b   The Safar airway.

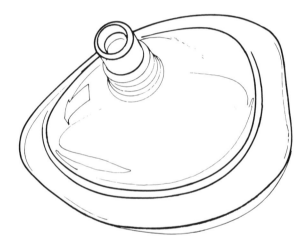

Fig. 8.2c.   The Laerdal mask.

The jaw of the victim needs to be supported properly with one hand, while the mask is held firmly in place at the same time, and the other hand is used to squeeze the bag. Inflation of the lungs should be observed and adjustment of the airway made if the chest is not seen to move on each inflation. If clumsily performed manual ventilation can result in inflation of the stomach. This is dangerous because smooth muscle tends to respond to the stretch stimulus by contraction, and gastric contents may then be expelled into the pharynx. Should the next inflation be properly performed, this material may be blown into the trachea and lungs.

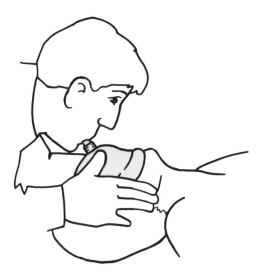

Fig. 8.2d.   The Laerdal mask in use.

Protection of the airway is provided by tracheal intubation with a cuffed tube.

Tracheal intubation (see Figs. 8.4–8.6)

The following account applies to any situation where this procedure may be required. The technique often appears to be very easy, and indeed it usually is to an expert, but sometimes it can be very difficult. The worst situation in which to have to perform tracheal intubation is when the patient is lying on the floor and in receipt of closed cardiac massage at the same time. The best situation in which to learn the principles of the manoeuvre is at the induction of general anaesthesia. These principles are the same whatever the indication for intubation.

1   The lungs should be inflated with oxygen up to the moment when laryngoscopy is started because, however expert the performance, it takes not less than 10 seconds to accomplish. Oxygen uptake in the tissues continues during this time and arterial oxygen tension declines. If there is any delay and in the absence of prior oxygenation, the arterial oxygen tension may decrease to about 6.6 kPa (50 mmHg).

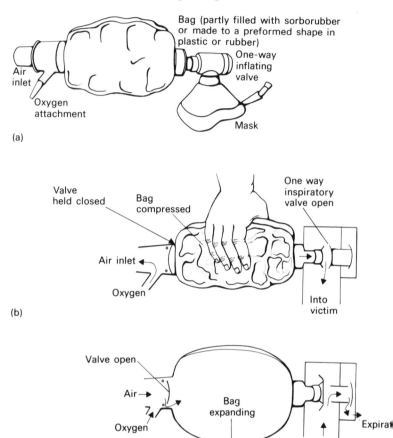

Fig. 8.3a A self-filling bag.
Fig. 8.3b & c Diagrams to illustrate the gas routes during use of a self-filling bag and inflating valve.

Oxygenation is not always possible during resuscitation from cardiac arrest but it should be attempted. Dysrhythmias occur as a result of both laryngoscopy and the passage of the tracheal tube through the larynx, and they are likely to be less serious if the patient is well oxygenated.
2 The head must be correctly positioned (see Fig. 8.4). When this is not done the manoeuvre is difficult. The mouth is not usually in the

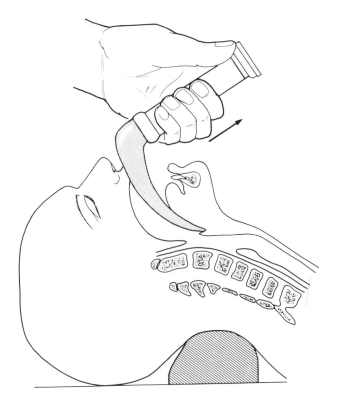

Fig. 8.4. The position of tip of laryngoscope blade and direction in which 'lift' should be applied. Note that the neck is flexed and the head extended at the atlanto-occipital joint.

same straight line as the laryngeal opening and the objective of the correct position is that they should be so manipulated. The neck (cervical spine) needs to be flexed and the head to be extended at the atlanto-occipital joint. This is usually achieved by a pillow under the neck at the level of lower cervical spine. The commonest error at this stage is to fail to remove the pillow from under, or behind, the shoulders. The position of the head and neck has been closely caricatured by the explanation 'it is like the position used when sniffing the morning air'.
3   The upper jaw is then pulled towards the operator with one finger and the lips pushed away from the teeth of the upper and lower jaws with the other fingers and thumb of the *right* hand (see Fig. 8.5). The

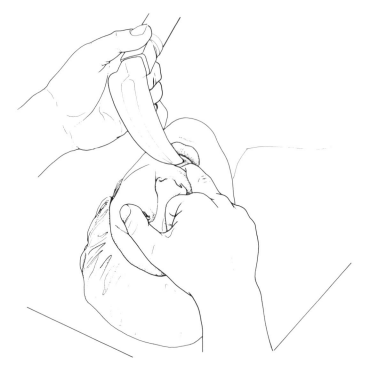

Fig. 8.5.   Introduction of laryngoscope.

muscles of the lower jaw need to be relaxed. Muscle relaxant drugs or general anaesthetic agents provide this; during cardiac arrest the jaws are usually relaxed sufficiently for laryngoscopy to be performed.

4   The laryngoscope is held in the *left* hand and introduced into the right side of the patient's mouth so that the tip of the laryngoscope blade approaches the midline from the right. This causes the tongue to be pushed out of the way and to the left. The design of the blade is such as to encourage this to happen.

5   The handle of the laryngoscope is then *lifted in the direction in which it points* (see Fig. 8.4). The teeth of the upper jaw, or the gums, must not be used as a fulcrum for a movement of rotation of the laryngoscope otherwise damage occurs both to them and to the delicate mucous membrane of the pharynx. The uvula can be seen at the tip of the blade

which is advanced in the midline whilst elevation of the soft tissues is maintained. The epiglottis is thus raised and the laryngeal opening is in view (see Fig. 8.6). The tip of the laryngoscope is now between the two pyriform fossae in the vallecula.

6 Intubation of the trachea is easy if the vocal cords are immobile in the cadaveric position. This is the case after muscle relaxants have been given. It is not so easy when cardiac massage is performed simultaneously and this should be stopped momentarily whilst the tracheal tube is passed through the cords. If the patient is making respiratory efforts at the same time the tube should be passed during inspiration when the cords are separated most widely.

7 Confirmation that the tube is correctly placed *must* now be sought. The chest may appear to move appropriately when the self-filling bag (or other reservoir bag), which is connected immediately is compressed

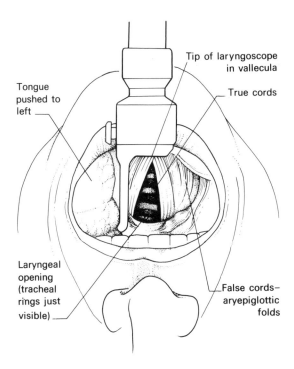

Fig. 8.6. Idealized view of larynx at laryngoscopy.

but this is not sufficient. Auscultation for breath sounds on both sides and in all areas of the chest must be performed and then, only if they are heard should the cuff of the tracheal tube be inflated.

8   The cuff is inflated with a sufficient volume of air so that leakage does not occur during inflation of the lungs.

Cardiac resuscitation

The term cardiac arrest is a generic one which includes the haemodynamic results of:

> asystole,
> ventricular fibrillation, or
> acute circulatory failure.

In two of these conditions cessation of contraction of the heart does not actually occur. When the output is so very low that all the signs of arrest are present as in circulatory failure it is certain that the heart will very shortly cease to function as a pump. In ventricular fibrillation there is no cardiac output, although incoordinate contraction of heart muscle continues.

The *diagnosis* of cardiac arrest is not always easy. The appearance of a dead body after the individual has been dead for a few minutes is characteristic. The skin is grey and pallid; it is cold to the touch and gravity-determined bluish mottling develops. If recovery is to be achieved there is not time to await the development of these changes.

The signs of cardiac arrest are:

> an absence of a previously palpable pulse, or
> an absence of pulsation of a major vessel (carotid or femoral).

Either one of these two cardinal signs is applicable in all situations.

It is necessary to make the diagnosis promptly within seconds of the event; otherwise treatment may be unavailing. Other important signs may follow and may deceive the unwary because they are not always present, detectable or diagnostic. Respiratory arrest, *apnoea*, may precede and usually follows cardiac arrest. *Unconsciousness* also usually develops. The measurement of *blood pressure* (which is unobtainable), *auscultation of the heart* (which is usually negative and requires that clothing be removed), the observation of an *electrocardiogram* (which, if not already attached, takes several minutes to apply) and *retinoscopy* (which requires an ophthalmoscope to be available to enable gaps in the columns of blood in blood vessels of the retina to be seen) are all unnecessary. If, of course, any or all of these variables are under observation at the critical moment they offer strong supporting evidence of the diagnosis, but otherwise vital seconds should not be wasted in an attempt to obtain them.

It is worth noting in this connection that when pressure is applied both sides of the neck on both carotid arteries the electroencephalograph takes at least 20 seconds to become flat, and that when total cardiopulmonary bypass is instituted the electrocardiogram may remain unchanged for as long as 60 seconds. The detection of one cardinal sign of cardiac arrest does not take longer than this and is preferable.

Pupillary dilatation follows circulatory arrest but this also occurs in atropine overdosage, or after surface application of the drug to the eye, and is a sign of hypoxia. Pupillary dilatation may not occur promptly in cases of morphine poisoning. The skin rapidly becomes *cyanosed*: this sign may not be so apparent in cases of carbon monoxide poisoning in which the blood is bright red and it occurs in many other conditions. Hypoxia may also precede the arrest and thus both cyanosis and mydriasis may already be present although the cardiac output is not impaired.

Why must treatment be immediate?

The basal oxygen requirement is about 250–300 ml per minute. Normally, although the arterial oxygen tension is about 13.3 kPa (100 mmHg), that in the middle of cells is much less than 1.3 kPa (10 mmHg). Cells at a greater distance from arterioles have lower oxygen tensions than those close to vessels and are probably at greater risk from hypoxia. A pressure gradient for oxygen is required in order for it to reach the cells and since mixed venous oxygen tension is usually about 6.6 kPa (50 mmHg) it is clear that there is not much margin for reduction. In chronic hypoxia (anaemia, high altitude etc.) various compensatory mechanisms are active, but these probably do not have time to develop in states of acute hypoxia.

There are no real reserves of oxygen in the body but at any one instant there is about 1000 ml of oxygen available.

Available oxygen = cardiac output × oxygen saturation
                          × haemoglobin concentration ×
                          haemoglobin carrying capacity for
                          oxygen,

$$\text{i.e. for adult man, } = 5000 \times \frac{99}{100} \times \frac{15}{100} \times 1.34$$

$$\approx 1000 \text{ ml/minute.}$$

Another estimate is of theoretical interest and emphasises the same point.

Body oxygen   = oxygen in the lungs + oxygen in blood
Oxygen in lungs = alveolar concentration × functional
                         residual capacity of lungs
                  ≈300 ml
Oxygen in blood = oxygen capacity × blood volume
(assume 30% blood volume is fully oxygenated and the remainder is 75% saturated)
                  ≈ 800 ml

It is obvious that not all this oxygen is fully available for metabolic purposes because it is neither delivered to the tissues nor can it diffuse to the cells because the pressure gradient is too small. Thus if oxygen uptake continues unabated the 'reserve' is utilized after, at most, 3 minutes. The inherent risks of pre-existing hypoxia are obvious and it is this fact which accounts for the observation that hypoxic patients withstand an episode of cardiac arrest poorly.

If the circulation does not restart spontaneously, or is not augmented artificially, within 3 minutes of the moment of its cessation, in general, it is probably unwise even to commence resuscitation. Cerebral damage is almost inevitable and gross neurological impairment may appear subsequently, even though cardiorespiratory function is adequate. The exceptions to this rule are young children, who withstand effects of cerebral hypoxia, or at least appear to, better than adults, and the presence of hypothermia, which reduces the cerebral demand and utilization of oxygen. There are case reports of full neurological recovery after cardiac arrest which lasted several minutes in both these circumstances.

Primary resuscitation

Technique of external cardiac compression (see Fig. 8.7).

1 The victim must lie on a firm surface. A single sharp blow on the precordium may restart normal cardiac action occasionally.

2 The sternum must be pushed towards the spine by about 5 cm each compression. Each compression should be a sharp defined

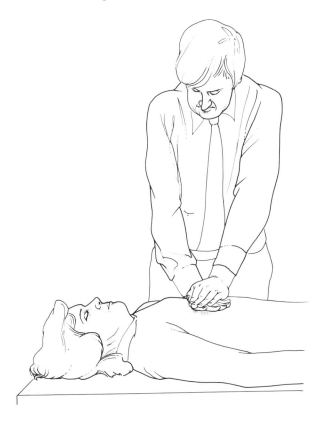

Fig. 8.7. External cardiac resuscitation.

movement performed at a rate of about 60–70 times per minute.

3 The heel of one of the rescuer's hands should be placed in the midline at the lower end of the sternum. The fingers must be kept clear of the chest wall and the other hand is superimposed upon the first.

Both arms should be straight.

The *efficacy* of the resuscitation should be assessed frequently by: feeling for a *pulse* in a major artery, and/or by observing the *pupil* size.

Further notes about external cardiac compression.

The object of external cardiac compression is that the heart should be compressed between the posterior surface of the sternum and the anterior surface of the dorsal vertebral bodies. The intracardiac valves determine the direction of the flow of blood.

Most of the weight of a man of average build is required to achieve the necessary movement of the sternum but even then less than half the normal stroke volume of the heart can be delivered.

In old victims it is almost inevitable that fractures of the ribs occur; indeed, it is sometimes stated that it is impossible to perform efficient external cardiac compression without such damage. Other direct damage to lungs, pericardium, aorta, liver and spleen is not an infrequent finding at subsequent autopsy.

If the pulse is felt just after each compression it may mean that blood is flowing but this must be distinguished from a fluid thrill which occurs in the absence of flow. There is always a thrill and other evidence may have to be sought of blood flow. If the pupil became dilated at the time of arrest it may now begin to constrict when blood flow is restored. The sign of capillary refill may return. On rare occasions the patient may regain consciousness.

Secondary cardiac resuscitation

Sometimes expired-air resuscitation and external cardiac compression are started by non-medical staff. This is all to the good because immediate treatment *is* vital. The next few minutes are important for the success of the therapy and the various tasks need to be carried out promptly, without panic, but as quickly and precisely as possible.

An *electrocardiogram* must be attached and the tracing examined to discern the reappearance of normal complexes and to enable the differential diagnosis to be made. Sometimes normal complexes are found at this stage and recriminative remarks passed, by doctors who should know better, to the effect that cardiac arrest cannot have occurred. This is unfortunate because no-one can be certain and it is better to perform resuscitation unnecessarily early than to delay until no technique can be successful.

An *intravenous infusion* must be established so that sodium bicarbonate can be administered to counteract the metabolic acidosis which is an inevitable consequence of circulatory arrest. If metabolic acidosis persists defibrillation may be ineffective or only temporarily effective. Approximate correction of metabolic acidosis with 100 mmol sodium bicarbonate should be made now. A sample of arterial blood for gas analysis should be obtained so that a check on hydrogen ion activity, oxygenation, and carbon dioxide elimination may be made.

It is usual but not essential at this stage to secure the airway by means of a tracheal tube. *Manual ventilation of the lungs with oxygen* is continued at a frequency of about 12 per minute in the pauses between each five or six external compressions of the heart; 100% oxygen is used because pulmonary oedema is a frequent result of both the arrest of the heart *and* of the resuscitation procedure. Diffusion of oxygen across the alveoli is improved if a marked concentration gradient exists.

Tertiary resuscitation

This includes defibrillation and drug therapy as indicated.

Asystole is treated by continued external cardiac compression, and adrenaline or isoprenaline may be given by intracardiac injection or via a large central vein, in an attempt to provoke coarse ventricular fibrillation. Electrical defibrillation of the heart often then results in restoration of sinus rhythm. Electrical pacing, on the other hand, is seldom successful in the resuscitation of a patient with asystolic cardiac arrest.

Ventricular fibrillation is treated by DC defibrillation. 100–400 joules are applied externally by the discharge of a previously charged capacitor.

Persistent *dysrhythmias* may require treatment with atropine, isoprenaline, lignocaine or disopyramide according to their nature. It may also be necessary to expand the blood volume.

Direct (internal) cardiac compression is seldom, if ever, indicated outside the operating room. It is conveniently performed during thoracotomy and, if the abdomen is already open the surgeon can, of course, compress the heart manually through the diaphragm, but otherwise immediate external, rather than internal, compression is indicated.

Further treatment

Late management after successful resuscitation may include treatment of pulmonary or cerebral oedema and respiratory, cardiac or renal failure. The genesis of pulmonary oedema has already been mentioned.

Cerebral oedema follows cerebral hypoxia. The signs may vary from:
  slow recovery of consciousness,
  inadequate ventilation,
  gasping, stertorous breathing,
  localized convulsions,
  rigidity,
  generalized convulsions,
  to prolonged coma.

Dehydration by intravenous hypertonic solutions, dexamethasone and hypothermia, combined with intermittent positive pressure ventilation are used in the attempt to reduce cerebral oedema and to reduce the demand for oxygen.

Causes of cardiac arrest

There is no single cause of cardiac arrest and many factors may be simultaneously or singly involved. Some of these factors become apparent after the event; others are obvious beforehand.

  Three common interacting and important factors are:
  hypoxia,
  hyperkalaemia, and
  hypercapnia.

Fig. 8.8 gives an outline of the interactions of these factors. Healthy patients withstand hypercapnia well; hypoxia or intercurrent disease, particularly of the heart, make the risks of hypercapnia serious. The importance of potassium in all these mechanisms can be seen. High concentrations of some inhaled anaesthetic drugs are irritant and initiate *vagal reflexes* as do a number of traction reflexes arising in the viscera. All these can cause cardiac asystole.

Catastrophic *haemorrhage* with the resultant decline in coronary perfusion also causes cardiac arrest. Many *other acute disasters* (massive pulmonary embolism, air embolus, overdose of cardioactive drugs, drowning or electrocution) may similarly cause cardiac arrest but the mechanisms at a cellular level can usually be related to hypoxia, hyperkalaemia or hypercapnia.

Results of resuscitation from cardiac arrest

If cardiac arrest occurs during an otherwise uncomplicated anaesthetic, in the recovery room, or in the intensive therapy unit, the results

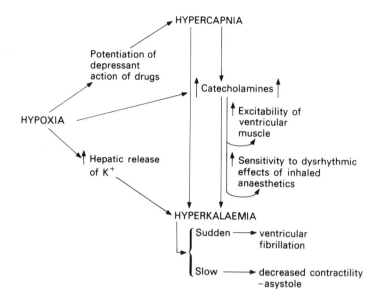

Fig. 8.8. Interactions between hypoxia, hypercapnia and hyperkalaemia.

of resuscitation should be better than those following resuscitation in other departments of the hospital or outside hospital. This is because both apparatus and skilled personnel are immediately available.

There are marked differences in the results which are claimed in the medical literature. Ventricular fibrillation carries a better prognosis than asystole. On the average about one third of the victims of cardiac arrest are resuscitated successfully in hospital but only about 12% are still alive one month after the incident. The long-term prognosis for young children is better than that for adults. The success rate in adults aged less than 40 years is less good than that for those over that age. This is partly, at least, due to the fact that an event sufficient to cause cardiac arrest in a patient less than 40 years old is probably itself catastrophic whereas that causative of arrest in an older patient may be less severe.

Cardiac arrest which happens after a long period of hypoxaemia is frequently terminal.

Ethics of cardiorespiratory resuscitation

This is a question much discussed by the lay public who often have views which are untenable by informed experts. It is important to remember that

> everyone must eventually die, and
> everyone has a right to a dignified death.

When cardiorespiratory arrest occurs resuscitation should always be attempted immediately by the first person on the scene. Subsequent arrivals may, because they are aware of other relevant medical details about the patient, elect to discontinue resuscitation. It is unlikely on the one hand, that a patient with widespread metastatic carcinoma should be allowed to undergo a strenuous attempt at resuscitation. On the other hand, a patient who has had one myocardial infarction should not be denied the benefits of resuscitation merely because a second infarction has caused cardiac arrest. It is dubious whether definitive decisions should ever be made in advance.

(Confusion also exists amongst the lay public between cardiorespiratory resuscitation, intensive therapy, and the ethics of organ transplantations. These subjects are not within the scope of this book.)

Resuscitation of the newborn

After delivery the neonate does not always begin spontaneous ventilation immediately and respiratory resuscitation may be required. The baby is placed supine on an open, heated incubator and slightly head down to encourage drainage of amniotic fluid; if there are any attempts at spontaneous ventilation an oxygen mask is held over the face. One minute after birth a rapid assessment is made of the:

> heart rate,
> respiratory effort,
> muscle tone,
> reflex irritability, and
> colour.

These five factors are scored and the Apgar system is widely employed to aid communication in this difficult field (Table 8.1). The ability to observe colour is so variable that it is often omitted and the total ideal score reduced to 8 instead of 10. The score at one minute after delivery does not distinguish between babies who have primary

Table 8.1 The Apgar scoring system

Apgar score	Heart rate	Respiratory effort	Muscle tone	Reflex irritability	Colour
0	Absent	Absent	Flaccid	Nil	White or blue
1	< 100/min	Hypo-ventilation Weak cry	Some limb flexion	Some movement	Cyanosed periphery
2	> 100/min	Normo-ventilation	Normal tone and all limbs flexed	Active	Pink

apnoea who will recover, and those who require active resuscitation if they are to survive. The picture is clearer by 5 minutes when the assessment is repeated.

If spontaneous ventilation is absent inflation of the lungs must be performed with a self-filling bag and mask designed especially for this use. Expired-air resuscitation can be used in primitive circumstances but otherwise the technique should be eschewed in neonates. Once the process of oxygenation has started, rhythmic ventilation may be established. If it is not, tracheal intubation should be performed. This procedure is not for the tyro since damage to delicate tissues and complete failure are often the only result of such attempts: manual ventilation using a bag and mask should be continued until skilled assistance is available.

When the trachea has been intubated tracheal suction can be performed and often a little mucus, meconium or amniotic fluid is removed. Adequate ventilation may then be followed by the onset of spontaneous respiration. Apnoea persists if the neonate is very premature or has suffered an intracranial haemorrhage during or immediately after delivery: artificial ventilation is then continued.

If cardiac arrest occurs external cardiac compression can be carried out with two fingers depressing the sternum. An artificial circulation can be maintained readily but even then permanent success is not guaranteed.

Respiratory stimulant drugs have no place in the management of the newly born. *Naloxone* is used to counteract respiratory depression caused by pethidine administered to the mother for analgesia prior to delivery.

Sodium bicarbonate may be required if resuscitation is delayed or if there is prolonged hypoxia which results in metabolic acidosis.

Resuscitation prior to emergency surgery

The term resuscitation is commonly applied to the preparation of a patient prior to emergency surgery. This preparation may include:

> intravenous fluids, including blood,
> analgesia, and
> oxygen therapy.

Another use of the term resuscitation is made particularly in European countries which have special emergency first aid services whose staff include anaesthetists, nurses and technicians. These teams attend industrial and road accidents and initiate early treatments (see Chapter 9). The principles of therapy are the same wherever it is to be carried out.

Resuscitation from haemorrhage

Haemorrhage may be:

> overt (e.g. haematemesis, open wounds), or
> covert (e.g. fractured bones, ruptured aneurysm or ectopic pregnancy)

The identification of the anatomical source of *overt* haemorrhage may not be so important at the time of the patient's presentation as are the assessment and management of the haemodynamic impairment. Reports and estimates of the volume lost are usually inadvertently exaggerated by onlookers but they should be noted.

Covert haemorrhage is paradoxically easier to assess because objective measurements of the girth of the abdomen or of a limb give some idea of the volume held within. For example, a closed fracture of the femur in an adult can result in the loss of as much as one litre of blood. Loss of double that volume may follow a closed fracture of the pelvis or multiple rib fractures. Summation of the volumes assessed by this means indicates the severity of the loss which may be sustained as a result of multiple injuries (Table 8.2).

The *clinical assessment* of the cardiovascular system of the injured patient is based on similar tests to those described in Chapter 7. The first response to haemorrhage is that of vasoconstriction. Catecholamine secretion is increased. Vasoconstriction has the effect of reducing skin

Table 8.2 Approximate blood loss in trauma

Number of major fractures	Blood loss (litres)
1	1
2	1-2
3	2-3

Additional losses occur when there are abdominal injuries also.

perfusion and causing pallor. The response is teleologically designed to promote perfusion of the brain at the expense of all other organs. The blood pressure may at this stage be normal or even elevated.

The lung suffers from reduced perfusion with the result that physiological dead space is increased considerably. Pain and shivering increase the tissue demand for oxygen and this, combined with the increased wastage of ventilation, causes the sign of air hunger. This is a typical sign of a patient who has bled considerably. If analgesics are given to suppress pain, it is likely that hypoxaemia will also develop unless, in addition, oxygen is administered.

Management. Fig. 8.9 shows the *posture* of a patient who has collapsed from any cause but particularly following haemorrhage. The legs are flexed at the hip joints. The trunk remains horizontal. If the head is also lowered any increase in cerebral blood flow is very temporary because flow is impeded by the back pressure of the column of blood in the jugular veins. Venous return is increased by the position shown in the Fig. 8.9 because blood is drained away from the legs. The benefits of this autotransfusion are lost if haemorrhage continues.

Analgesic drugs should be administered intravenously. Blood flow to muscles is decreased and absorption from intramuscular sites may be very delayed. Small doses of analgesics should be given repeatedly until a satisfactory effect is achieved.

Oxygen should be given.

Intravenous infusions should be established in large veins with large bore cannulae as soon as possible.

The flow of fluid through a cannula is determined predominantly by its internal diameter. The height of the transfusion reservoir above the vein, that is, the driving pressure, is of less importance. Doubling the radius of the cannula theoretically increases the flow through it by a

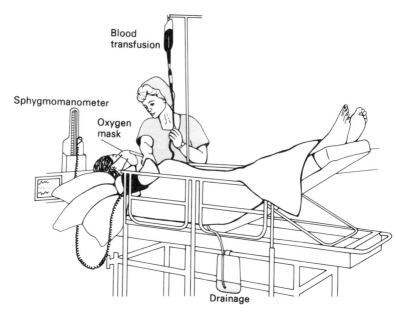

Fig. 8.9. Posture of a patient who is bleeding actively following operation. Note that the legs are raised at the hips but the remainder of the body is kept horizontal.

factor of 16 but doubling the height of the reservoir above the cannula only doubles the flow.

In practice the increases are much less than this because the physical law (Poisieuille) governing these relationships applies precisely to streamline or laminar flow. Large volume flow rates through narrow gauge channels result in turbulence and the law does not apply. Table 8.3 shows a few figures which illustrate this point. Note that the length of the cannula is a relatively unimportant factor in determining flow rate: a long catheter impedes volume flow but not by a great amount. Viscous solutions (blood) flow more slowly than non-viscous ones (saline). The gauge of the cannula is clearly a dominant factor in the determination of volume flow rates.

The choice of fluid to be infused depends on the magnitude of the estimated loss. After massive loss the nature of the fluid is unimportant and any expansion of the circulating volume is beneficial. It is usual to commence with the nearest solution to hand which is often a crystalloid such as Ringer's lactate (Hartmann's). This remains in the circulation

Table 8.3 Relative importance of dimensions of cannulae in determining flow rate

Length (mm)	Inside diameter (mm)	Flow of water (ml/min)
*Type 1**		
47	1.45	275
47	1.2	175
47	1.0	115
47	0.8	75
47	0.6	35
Type 2†		
57	1.4	218
89	1.4	210
140	1.4	196

* Manufacturers' data.
† From Bell, G.T. & Farman, J.V. (1972) *British Journal of Hospital Medicine,* Equipment Supplement **8,** 49.

briefly; massive transfusions with electrolyte solutions confer no permanent benefit and may do frank harm. The blood pressure may rise temporarily or not at all. Colloid solutions (dextran 70, starch or gelatin solutions) remain in the circulation for longer periods. Plasma preparations (plasma protein fraction or fresh frozen plasma) are possible alternatives which are more similar to the fluid which has been lost than the above synthetic ones. The real answer is, of course, blood transfusion but (apart from universal donor blood Group O Rh.—ve) transfusions must be crossmatched and this may take time.

If surgery is to be immediate and is likely to result in further haemorrhage such as, for example, in patients with ruptured aortic aneurysms, monitoring lines (urinary catheter, central venous and arterial pressure) should also be established. In some centres these patients are wrapped in an abdominal pressure suit which prevents further loss from the aorta and enables resuscitation to be carried out without panic.

The precise timing of surgery may be a matter for nice judgement. Where blood loss has been finite and has ceased it is clear that operation can be performed as soon as the loss appears to have been replaced. Blood loss is often continuous and may even be aggravated by resuscitation. If the patient continues to improve there should be no rush to commence operation. When, however, improvement ceases or deterioration occurs in spite of energetic resuscitation then surgery must start promptly. Resuscitation continues during surgery although general anaesthesia itself may contribute to the urgency of treatment.

Resuscitation from dehydration

Dehydration is a serious result of many general surgical emergencies and occurs as a result of:

  starvation,
  aspiration of stomach contents without replacement,
  vomiting,
  intestinal obstruction,
  perforated viscus,
  intestinal fistulae, or
  diarrhoea.

The *clinical diagnosis* of dehydration depends on the presence of a history of one of the above conditions and its associated physical signs, and the detection of a few clinical signs of dehydration. The skin loses its elasticity and does not readily recover its normal shape after it has been pinched. The tongue is dry and furred; halitosis may be marked. Intraocular tension is low and the eyeball is often frankly soft.

Laboratory tests confirm these observations. Urine output is low, its specific gravity and its osmolarity are high. The haemoglobin is raised and so is the haematocrit. Blood urea is also raised. The serum electrolyte levels reflect the losses if they have been severe. There may be metabolic alkalosis or acidosis. Prolonged vomiting is associated with metabolic alkalosis and hypokalaemia. Potassium ions migrate into cells in place of lost hydrogen ions. Severe continued intestinal obstruction results in metabolic acidosis due to hypovolaemia.

Management aims to correct these losses with appropriate fluids. Thus patients who have lost sodium and potassium, as a result of diarrhoea or an intestinal fistula, are treated with infusions of saline (rarely more concentrated than 0.9%) with additional potassium as potassium chloride.

Treatment when there is a metabolic derangement should be directed to the primary cause. It is seldom necessary to treat the metabolic disturbance specifically prior to emergency surgery. Appropriate intravenous fluids, assuming there is unimpaired renal function, are all that is necessary at this stage.

When perforation of an abdominal viscus is suspected it is likely that widespread inflammation with loss of protein-rich fluid will develop. The use of colloid solutions, particularly plasma, during emergency resuscitation rather than crystalloid solutions is claimed to counteract the development of tissue oedema.

Technique of intravenous injection

Unconscious patients complain less than conscious ones and opportunities to practise under ideal conditions should be sought. Large needles are not necessary for intravenous injections, and when very fine needles are used even conscious patients are often unaware that an injection has been made.

Any visible vein *can* be punctured but it is better to avoid vessels which are very close to the known, or presumed, course of arteries. Intra-arterial injections of many drugs cause permanent undesirable sequelae. The skin of the antecubital fossa is less sensitive than that at the wrist or dorsal surface of the hand. The medial side of the antecubital fossa is particularly dangerous because the brachial artery lies superficially.

Veins are anchored to the deep fascia at junctions. Junctions are therefore suitable sites for intravenous injections. The skin should be cleaned with antiseptic and then punctured a short distance from the proposed point of entry into the vein (see Fig. 8.10). This limits the

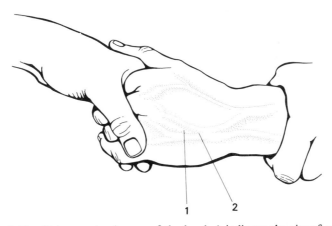

Fig. 8.10. Veins on the dorsum of the hand. 1 indicates the site of entry through the skin when puncture at site 2, at the junction of two veins, is proposed.

subsequent spread of any haematoma and also tends to prevent transfixion of the vein. The needle is then slid along the course of the vein to prevent it from cutting out, aspiration of blood into a syringe confirms success and the injection can be given. The needle is held in place with the thumb of one hand whilst the fingers grasp the limb or hand (Fig. 8.11). If the patient were to move, or attempt to move, the needle can be held firmly in place whilst the patient does not have to be immobile. The other hand is used to perform the injection.

The same vein can be used repeatedly for injection if care is taken when the needle is removed and particularly if a fine needle is used. Firm pressure over the site and elevation of the limb to avoid venous distension is all that is required.

Technique of intravenous cannulation

The antecubital fossa is an inappropriate site for an intravenous infusion because of the severe restriction of movement which is thereby imposed. In general it is desirable to arrange that the cannula, once in place, should not itself come to rest over a joint. If it does, whatever the method of fixation, it will soon come out of the vein.

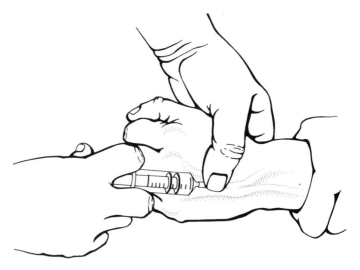

Fig. 8.11. Thumb position of one hand when holding the hub of the needle in place during an injection.

Local analgesia (0.25 ml 1% lignocaine) at the site of puncture makes the procedure almost painless.

The technique of insertion of a cannula is very similar to injection, but instead of sliding the needle along the vein the cannula is passed over the trocar (needle) and since this is usually blunt-ended there is much less risk of further damage to the vein.

Not all cannulae can be used easily through the intact skin, and the tips of some tend easily to curl back on the trocar. These should be discarded. A small cut (about 1–2 mm long) can be made in the skin to enable the cannula to be passed easily.

The cannula must be attached to the patient's skin with an adhesive strapping to which no known allergy exists. If the site has been chosen correctly, and the insertion performed in a careful and sterile manner with a modern plastic cannula, intravenous infusions can be maintained for long periods.

9. A miscellany of special topics

This chapter is devoted to a series of brief comments on unconnected special topics related to anaesthesia which are of general interest to undergraduate medical students.

Specialization

There has been considerable specialization amongst anaesthetists with the result that significant progress has been achieved in several fields. Most specialties of surgery have their own unique problems which are the concern of a few surgical specialists. Many aspects of anaesthesia in these specialties are no different from those of any other apart from a few which are worthy of comment. Cooperation between all members of the team seems to improve the therapeutic effectiveness of the individuals within the team. Furthermore, this approach to problems often produces benefits in both research and development.

Thoracic surgery would not have progressed to the extent that it has today without the interest of anaesthetists who sought a solution to the problem posed by the open thorax. Spontaneous ventilation under these circumstances is not only ineffective but it is also frankly harmful: the mediastinum tends to move with the movements of ventilation with a resultant undesirable decrease in venous return. This is caused by direct compression of the vena cava but, in addition, the thoracic pump mechanism is abolished immediately the thoracic cavity is open and the subatmospheric pressure therein is lost. It was early appreciated that controlled ventilation (manual) was the solution to this problem and this was accomplished first with ether, then with cyclopropane, and later with the aid of muscle relaxants. Machines were soon developed to ventilate the lungs automatically; the anaesthetist's hands were thus freed from the performance of manual ventilation and the era of unhurried intrathoracic surgery commenced. Cardiac surgery and the entire practice of intensive therapy were natural and inevitable developments: furthermore, successful cardiac surgery depends on postoperative intensive therapy.

Another problem posed by surgical operations upon diseased lungs (pulmonary tuberculosis or bronchiectasis) was the need to prevent the extension of disease by direct infection of hitherto unaffected lung. This was achieved by selective blockage of bronchi or by the use of bronchial tubes with single or double lumina. These techniques are not routinely required so frequently today as they were 20 years ago: nevertheless, intrapulmonary haemorrhage following bronchoscopy, surgery or accident can often be managed by these methods.

Intracardiac surgery, particularly the replacement of incompetent valves, correction of congenital malformations and revascularization procedures for ischaemic heart disease, demands team work of the highest order. Pulmonary function is taken over by an artificial oxygenator and the heart is entirely bypassed, so that the brain and other organs can continuously be supplied with oxygenated blood. This technique of cardiopulmonary bypass is often managed by anaesthetists in addition to their other responsibilities. The lungs are not ventilated during bypass, and so anaesthetic drugs must be given intravenously or added to the gas mixture (oxygen and carbon dioxide) supplied to the oxygenator.

One of the main benefits to have accrued from the advances in cardiac surgery is the understanding of acute haemodynamics in very ill patients. Invasive monitoring of vascular pressures is essential and, whilst the cardiac patients themselves have obviously benefited, this benefit has spread to the management of any very sick patient which has enormously improved as a result.

Neurosurgical anaesthesia is another field in which specialization by anaesthetists has been particularly beneficial. The patient's airway is relatively inaccessible to the anaesthetist after the operation has begun. Intracranial surgical procedures tend to be very prolonged and are often technically very demanding on the surgeon.

Hypothermia is used, both to reduce the bulk of the brain and to protect areas of brain from hypoxia should it be necessary to interrupt the blood supply during the operation. Haemorrhage, if it occurs, may be very difficult to control because of the limited access.

The size and tension of the intracranial contents may be reduced or increased by various events under the control of the anaesthetist. On the one hand, hyperventilation, induced hypotension and hypothermia may all be employed to improve surgical access. Hyperventilation reduces the volume of intracranial contents by causing a reduction in the arterial carbon dioxide tension. This, in turn, results in a decrease in cerebral blood flow. Induced hypotension may be used to assist the handling of an aneurysm. Ganglion blockade, sodium nitroprusside, halothane and muscular paralysis are common methods of achieving arterial hypotension.

Faulty anaesthetic techniques which result in coughing or straining, on the other hand, cause an increase in intracranial volume. Hypercapnia, hypoxia and many inhaled anaesthetic drugs cause increases in cerebral blood flow and thus increase the volume of the intracranial contents.

Air embolus is always possible since the venous sinuses are open to the atmosphere and a subatmospheric pressure can cause air to enter the circulation. Positive-positive pressure ventilation of the lungs and direct application of pressure to the jugular veins are employed at times of greatest risk. Ultrasonic detectors are placed over the precordium. Centrally placed venous catheters can sometimes be used to aspirate the air before it reaches the coronary vessels and causes cardiac arrest.

Neurosurgical operations are associated with considerable postoperative surgical morbidity; recovery is not always immediate or complete. Facilities for long-term intensive therapy are essential. Much of our understanding of coma has sprung from experience in neurosurgical intensive therapy units.

In similar ways, but perhaps less dramatically, teams for other specialties within surgery have developed and where Health Service needs dictate, special centres have been established in which teams for each type of surgery are concentrated.

Day case surgery

Economic pressures have resulted in the development of day case units for many superficial (non-cavity) operations. The benefits to the community are well recognized. The patient does not require to be admitted to an expensive hospital bed, returns home soon after operation and is visited there by the community nurse and general practitioner if necessary. If the patient is a child, family life is less disturbed than when admission to hospital is necessary and, it is claimed, behaviour disturbances are therefore less frequent.

Many operations can be performed under local analgesia and have been for many years. It is the provision of general anaesthesia in day units which has increased during the last few years. Certain safeguards are essential. Poor risk or elderly patients are not treated as day patients. The old are less well able to adapt quickly to changes and the steady, if slower, processes of inpatient care are more appropriate. Complications are more likely in both these groups and in the event are more conveniently managed in hospital. There must, in any case, always be provision for admission of a patient into hospital should the need arise.

When patients are seen by the anaesthetist prior to their arrival in the anaesthetic room, compliance with the request to starve overnight must be confirmed. A similar preoperative assessment to that for any other patient must be made.

It is advisable that general instructions be given in writing as well as verbally. These include the following warnings, that for 24 hours following a general anaesthetic, the recipient should not:

drive,

drink alcohol,

cook,

operate machinery, or

travel alone.

Each of these warnings is important. Patients often disregard them but they do so at no little risk. Anaesthetic drugs are present in the body for many hours after their effects appear to have ceased; slower than normal reaction times and faulty judgement are two undesirable features which may still operate and cause accidents. The effects of alcohol added to the residual effects of anaesthetic drugs can be profound. Memory and manipulative skills are also impaired for a long time after a general anaesthetic.

The patients are discharged from hospital when they have recovered from the anaesthetic and must be accompanied home by a responsible adult. Ambulances may have to be used although they are not essential. Arrangements can be made for a community nurse to visit the patient at home to check the state of any surgical wound and to administer appropriate analgesics. A second visit the following morning is all that is normally required.

Dental surgery in general dental practitioner surgeries has also been practised for many years and is a special form of day case surgery. It is now recognized that teeth extraction and conservation work should be performed only when two properly qualified people are present: one performs dentistry and the other, a professional medical anaesthetist or dentist trained in anaesthesia, administers the general anaesthetic. The patient should be horizontal. Acute cardiovascular collapse, not unlike a vasovagal faint, can lead to cardiac arrest. The horizontal position prevents this. The dental surgery should be equipped with equipment for resuscitation, oxygen and suction. Those who give anaesthetics in the dental surgery should be properly trained so to do.

Obstetrics

There are three parts of an anaesthetist's work in obstetric units: analgesia, anaesthesia and resuscitation of the new-born.

Analgesia during labour was for many years a somewhat haphazard affair. Routines were employed by obstetricians with scant knowledge and who were seldom present at normal deliveries and whose instructions were followed or interpreted by midwives. The efficacy of the treatment was unknown.

New drugs, technological improvements and social pressures have led anaesthetists to specialize in this field. Hypnosis, parenteral drugs, (usually sedatives and analgesics), self-administered nitrous oxide or trichloroethylene and regional analgesia (epidural or caudal usually, spinal rarely) are all used. Mothers can be offered a choice although this implies more understanding than can really exist. More than one method can be tried if the first one fails.

Anaesthesia may be merely an extension of an effective analgesic technique so that instrumental delivery may be employed, but general anaesthesia is commonly chosen. There may be little time for preparation of the patient and thus when labour begins in any patient she is only allowed small amounts of fluid orally. If forceps or Caesarean section are anticipated all oral fluids are stopped and antacid therapy is administered because:

> gastric contents are very acid,
> regurgitation is common in patients with distended abdomens,
> intragastric pressure is raised, and
> hiatus hernia is common.

Oral antacids are given every 2 hours and immediately before induction of general anaesthesia. Histamine antagonists are sometimes used for the same purpose. In the absence of these preparations the stomach may need to be emptied by other means. Haemorrhage is occasionally torrential and facilities for rapid blood transfusion are immediately available.

General anaesthesia is induced with the patient's loin supported with a wedge to prevent the inferior vena cava from compression (see p. 111). An assistant performs cricoid pressure as soon as consciousness is lost. This manoeuvre causes the oesophagus to be compressed by the backward movement of the cricoid cartilage and thus passive regurgitation of stomach contents into the trachea is prevented (see later). Central depressant drugs are kept to a minimum in order to avoid neonatal depression. Ventilation is controlled carefully to ensure oxygenation and to avoid hyperventilation: hypocapnia reduces splanchnic, and thus uterine, blood flow. In other respects the conduct of anaesthesia is similar to that for any other abdominal surgery.

Neonatal resuscitation (see Chapter 8) is part of many obstetric anaesthetists' work but it is of particular interest to paediatricians who also supervise it in some centres.

Anaesthetic outpatients

A few anaesthetic departments run an outpatient session to enable all patients to be seen about their anaesthetic before admission. This arrangement should ideally solve a number of problems, but in practice this does not seem to happen. Chapter 2 emphasises the value of personal contact between patient and anaesthetist. It is impractical, not to say unnecessary, to arrange for this to occur in outpatients for every patient but it may occasionally be required in unusual circumstances.

A similar approach is to arrange that necessary investigations are performed on patients who are seen shortly before admission – the preadmission clinic – in order to reduce hospital stay. This has no particular advantage for anaesthetists except that the results of relevant tests are available before surgery.

Pain clinics are a special and recent development of out-patient and in-patient work. A group of different specialists, usually including some of the following: neurologist, psychiatrist, radiotherapist, neurosurgeon, general physician, clinical pharmacologist and anaesthetist, all combine together to manage painful conditions which otherwise may be neglected or treated ineffectively.

The details of organization depend entirely on local circumstances. At one extreme, several hospital beds may be allocated to one doctor solely for this purpose and, at the other, the group of pain specialists may merely function within an internal cross-referral system.

Mild to moderate analgesics, combined with sedatives or psychotropic drugs which potentiate them, may be used. Pain tract surgery, pituitary ablation or other neurosurgical procedures are sometimes possible. The management of pain can certainly not be achieved by one specialist unless substantial time and effort are given. Equally, it is certain that the regional analgesic techniques with local anaesthetics, narcotics, alcohol or phenol, which anaesthetists may employ, sometimes effectively, are not the sole answer.

There are many patients in Hospices for the dying who would benefit from proper management of their pain: too many patients with advanced malignancy are given narcotic drugs in large doses and then allowed to die in a comatose state as if this were the only alternative to excruciating pain. Much more could be done to alleviate terminal pain and further study is needed.

Emergency operations

There are several important practical aspects of anaesthesia for emergency surgery. The fact that the operation is called an emergency means that without it the patient's life may be in jeopardy. The standards of care under these circumstances should not be any less than those for elective surgery although it is clear (see Chapter 2) that the risk is increased.

Preoperative *assessment* and preparation, both physical and psychological, has to be completed in a short time and may therefore be less than ideal. Less is known and less can be done about the patient's general physical state. *Dehydration* may be present and hypovolaemia must be, at least partially, corrected before general anaesthesia is induced (see Chapter 8).

The *full stomach* poses important problems before general anaesthesia. Retrograde emptying

> by passive regurgitation, or
> by active vomiting

may occur. If this happens the risk is that stomach contents may be able to enter the trachea and cause asphyxiation immediately or lobar collapse later.

The stomach may be full because of:

> a recent meal,
> delayed gastric emptying as a result of pain,
> intestinal obstruction or ileus.

Notwithstanding competent attempts to empty the stomach of solid material, there are circumstances (obstetrics, hiatus hernia or obesity) in which gastric acid aspiration into the lungs may happen in spite of the stomach being empty of food. Acid aspiration pneumonitis is a life-threatening condition and requires aggressive intensive therapy if a fatal outcome is to be avoided.

Preoperative management. Adequate stomach emptying is achieved prior to elective surgery by the simple, if sometimes inhumane, expedient of starvation. Many so-called emergencies (fractures, abscesses, wound debridement) can be delayed a few hours so that there is an interval of 6 hours after the last meal or 4 hours after the last drink. This regimen is widely adopted.

Urgent emergencies (bowel or limb salvage, active haemorrhage) cannot be delayed and mechanical methods of emptying the stomach must be employed. A fine Ryle's tube is useless: clear fluid may be aspirated but nothing more viscous than water can be removed from the stomach. A larger bore oesophageal tube may be more effective. Either of the former tubes or a wide bore stomach tube may cause the patient actively to vomit. None of these methods confers immunity from the serious hazards of a full stomach.

Two drugs should be mentioned here. Firstly, *apomorphine*, a drug which causes active vomiting is occasionally employed. It is unpleasant, promptly effective during intravenous administration and evanescent. It is quickly reversed by atropine.

Secondly, *metoclopramide* which is an antiemetic with phenothiazine-like action on the chemoreceptor trigger zone and also causes an increase in the speed with which the stomach empties. Metoclopramide has some sedative action and occasionally causes signs of Parkinsonism: its actions, apart from that on the chemoreceptor trigger zone, are antagonized by atropine.

Management and induction of general anaesthesia varies widely but the aim is always to protect the trachea with a tracheal tube. The choice includes a variety of postures and methods of induction; it is also possible to insert a tracheal tube while the patient is still conscious.

Posture may be: supine with 30° head up which increases the gradient against which stomach contents must flow or 30° head down which aids drainage of regurgitated material. The left lateral position also improves drainage so that material tends to flow out of the mouth rather than into the larynx.

Induction may be by inhalation with spontaneous ventilation actively maintained by additional carbon dioxide. This is effective since vomiting occurs during apnoea, which is prevented, but no particular protection is afforded against regurgitation. Regurgitation is hindered by the application of *cricoid pressure* on the oesophagus during loss of consciousness. An assistant grasps the cricoid cartilage between his index finger and thumb and pushes the cartilage backwards onto the oesophagus. Swift tracheal intubation follows. An alternative popular method involves preoxygenation for 5–10 minutes (although this is longer than required provided that the patient takes deep breaths), it is followed by a predetermined dose of a rapidly acting intravenous agent, cricoid pressure and muscle paralysis to aid rapid intubation of the trachea. It may be dangerous to inflate the lungs using a bag and mask if there is any delay in intubation because further distension of the stomach with air is almost inevitable and may result in contraction of the stomach and regurgitation. Local anaesthesia of the larynx and intubation before general anaesthesia is induced is used in some centres but this involves the serious risk that if the local is inadequate for intubation the trachea is nevertheless unprotected.

Regional anaesthesia is seldom the preferred solution to the problem of the full stomach because should anaesthesia be in any way inadequate, supplemental systemic sedation brings all the risks of general anaesthesia. The treatment of toxic effects of local anaesthetic drugs may also necessitate general anaesthesia and tracheal intubation.

Recovery from emergency anaesthesia is also a hazardous period since the risk of aspiration is still present. There is a little evidence to suggest that after general anaesthesia and tracheal intubation the laryngeal reflexes remain incompetent for several hours. Most anaesthetists aim, therefore, to have the patient awake and coughing prior to extubation of the trachea. This procedure is performed carefully, gently and swiftly with the patient in the lateral position (and commonly head down).

Other professional activities of anaesthetists

This book has emphasised the intellectual aspects of anaesthesia in relation to the understanding of physiology and pharmacology. The application of this knowledge led naturally to the practice of intensive therapy, pain relief in obstetrics and work in pain clinics. There are a few other para-anaesthetic subjects which must be mentioned.

Hypnosis is by no means the sole prerogative of anaesthetists although many find it a useful additional method in their practice. Obstetric patients have been helped by hypnosis but in general the method is too time-consuming. A few patients can be hypnotized to a level at which superficial operations can be performed.

Acupuncture analgesia has been used in a few Western pain clinics with satisfactory results. In general, since understanding of the mechanism is so meagre, medically qualified anaesthetists have been loth to experiment with the technique. Oriental patients do, however, undergo quite extensive superficial operations performed under acupuncture anaesthesia. There is no muscle relaxation. The author is unaware of any particular enthusiasm for this method in the United Kingdom.

Resuscitation at accidents outside hospital is a very new field of activity for anaesthetists. The concept is, however, well developed in some other European countries and is similar to that underlying the use of coronary ambulances. It is claimed that worthwhile resuscitation with intravenous fluids, analgesics, oxygen and airway supervision can be provided to victims at the site of an accident and that anaesthetists are naturally the specialists who should undertake this work. The techniques have been described earlier and this matter is currently under debate. It is perhaps worth noting that self-administration of analgesia (nitrous oxide, 50% in oxygen) by conscious patients who are in pain, which has proved an undoubted boon, was pioneered by an advocate of anaesthetists' attendance at accidents.

Appendix: some definitions and reference values

Boyle's law

At any given temperature the volume of a fixed mass of gas varies inversely as its pressure.

Strictly, this law applies to ideal gases: it is applied to real gas and the minor descrepancies which result are small enough to be ignored.

Dalton's law of partial pressures

In a mixture of gases, contained in a given volume at a given temperature, the total pressure of the mixture is equal to the sum of those pressures which the gases would exert if they were to exist separately in the same volume and at the same temperature.

Tidal volume (Vt)

This is the volume of gas in each breath and is usually measured in cubic centimetres (cm^3); $7\ cm^3 kg^{-1}$ is a normal value for a spontaneously breathing conscious adult; $10\text{-}12\ cm^3 kg^{-1}$ is a common value for controlled ventilation under anaesthesia at a frequency of 12 per minute.

Minute volume ($\dot{V}E$)

This is the total volume of ventilation per minute. Expired minute ventilation is usually measured hence the subscript E.

It is the product of tidal volume and respiratory frequency (f, breaths per minute). It is usually measured in litres per minute (or $dm^3\ min^{-1}$).

Alveolar ventilation (VA)

This is the minute volume of ventilation which actually exchanges gases in the alveoli. It is less than the total ventilation by a volume called the physiological dead space. The volume of the physiological dead space is about one third of that of the total minute volume in a conscious erect young man: it is increased by anaesthesia, with increasing age, by other physiological events and pathological processes.

Vital capacity

This is the volume of the largest expiration after a maximal inspiration. Its value depends upon height, ethnic background, physical fitness, smoking history and gender. The accompanying table shows values for men.

	Vital capacity (dm^3, or litres)		
Height cm 170 (5′7″)	4.8	4.5	3.7
175 (5′9″)	5.1	4.7	4.0
180 (5′11″)	5.3	5.0	4.2
Age (yrs)	20	35	70

Forced expiratory volume in 1 second ($FEV_{1.0}$)

This is the volume of gas expired in one second. In normal subjects without lung disease it is more than 75% of the vital capacity. When it is less than 60—65%, pathological narrowing of the airways exists.

Atmospheric air (dry)

	Concentration	Partial pressure	
	volumes %	kPa	mmHg
Oxygen	20.95	21.20	159
Nitrogen	78.09	79.10	590
Carbon dioxide	0.03	0.03	0.23
Inert gases	0.93	0.93	7
	100.00	101.26	756.23

Alveolar gas

	Concentration	Partial pressure	
	volumes %	kPa	mmHg
Oxygen	13.4	13.5	102
Carbon dioxide	4.8	4.9	37
Nitrogen	75.5	76.3	574
Water vapour	6.2	6.2	47
	99.9	100.9	760

Systeme Internationale Units (SI)

The similarity between the numbers representing concentration of gases (%) and partial pressures in kiloPascals (kPa) should be noted. For most clinical purposes atmospheric pressure can be assumed to be 100 kPa and therefore alveolar carbon dioxide of 4.8% concentration exerts a partial pressure of 4.8 kPa.

Calculation of a partial pressure from a concentration

For example, there is 20.95% oxygen in the atmosphere.
   Total barometric pressure at sea level
   $= 760$ mmHg
Therefore
   Partial pressure of oxygen (from Dalton's Law)
   $$= \frac{20.95}{100} \times 760$$
   $$= 159 \text{ mmHg}$$
When the SI system is used this calculation is not necessary.

Blood gas tensions

	Arterial		Venous	
	kPa	mmHg	kPa	mmHg
Oxygen	13.3	100	5.3	40
Carbon dioxide	5.3	40 (36—44)	6.1	46
	(4.8—5.8)			

Arterial oxygen tension (PaO_2) is related to age in years

$$PaO_2 = 104 - \frac{Age}{4} \text{ mmHg}$$

or, $14 - \dfrac{Age}{30}$ kPa

Index

169